A disease called
Fatigue

by
Cécile Jadin

A disease called
Fatigue

by
Cécile Jadin

Foreword by
Tim Roberts (Assoc.Professor)

Faculty of Science and Information Technology,
School of Environmental and Life Sciences,
University of Newcastle Assistant Dean (International)
Chairperson Bio-molecular Research Facility Committee,
University of Newcastle Australia.

Published by hph Publishing

Science Rosier
English version First Edition
Cover illustration: Cécile Jadin
www.chronicfatiguesyndrome.tv
Private bag X 153, suite 33,
Bryanston 2021 South Africa
Copyright 2002
ISBN: 0-620-29265-2

To Juno

CONTENTS

FOREWORD

It is not often in one's lifetime that one meets such a remarkable human being as Cecile Louise Jadin - a successful artist, a brilliant clinician, a wonderful wife and mother, and a compassionate and visionary person. Her life experiences range from the jungles of the Congo, through the art scene of Paris and the Medical School of the University of Louvain, Belgium, to her specialisation in surgery and, finally, to clinical practice in South Africa.

In this book she gives an insight into some of her attributes, as she outlines her impressive contribution to modern medicine. She reminds us all that it is not possible to successfully look at human health by following the silo approach of the medical specialist. Her unique understanding of the manifold symptomatology of chronic rickettsial infection has allowed her to successfully diagnose and treat patients, who (depending on which specialty was present at the final diagnosis) were classified as having chronic fatigue syndrome, depression, schizophrenia, autism, auto-immune disease or heart disease.

In her childhood and teenage years, Cecile witnessed the wondrous scientific discoveries of intracellular infectious bacteria made by her father, Professor J B Jadin. In tropical medicine, he and his colleagues had pioneered the understanding of the role of those microbes, which had evolved life cycles midway between free-living bacteria and viruses. Unfortunately for the English-speaking world, the bulk of his many scientific publications have remained relatively inaccessible in French language medical journals.

Although initially choosing to follow an artist's life, Cecile eventually enrolled to study medicine, and then specialised in surgery. Such a progression was natural for the medical student of the seventies, as medicine had become the science of distinct silos or specialisation. The endocrinologist dealt with hormones, the immunologist with auto-immunity, the psychiatrist with mental illness, and so on.

Cecile resisted the urge to adopt her father's work and findings into her medicine, but when in her practice she continually saw chronically ill patients who had failed to have their illnesses cured by specialists – patients with a plethora of disease symptoms with no defined etiological agents – she began to suspect that the intracellular infections which had been the passion of her father – the rickettsias and the chlamydias - were really at the root of these symptoms. Cecile began testing these patients with the micro agglutination test developed by her father, to detect antibodies against rickettsia, and the findings were positive. She then instituted a regime of antibiotic treatment based on that developed by her father, and the results have been spectacular.

Cecile found that she was able to treat successfully these chronically-diseased individuals, who because of the length of their infection had been classified as psychiatric patients, malingerers, or sufferers of chronic pain, chronic fatigue syndrome or irritable bowel syndrome.

She has enjoyed remarkable success in treating these patients over the past 10 years, whilst enduring considerable opposition as she came up against the medical establishment in the guise of the South African Doctors' Registration Board. For four years she was engaged in a constant battle to prove that her treatment methods were indeed effective. This book is a delightful and inspirational account of her philosophy of medicine. She reminds us of the lessons to be learnt from history and the importance of dedication to a belief in one's self.

Tim Roberts
Associate Professor, Faculty of Science and Information Technology, School of Environmental and Life Sciences, University of Newcastle; Assistant Dean (International); Chairperson Bio-molecular Research Facility Committee, University of Newcastle; Member of Editorial Board of the Journal of Chronic Fatigue Syndrome.

PREFACE

Our more refined, careful knowledge is only an infinite fragment when it is compared to the cosmos. Medicine, history and politics force themselves in a similar way through time and space to gather all the various phenomena and the extreme variety of their content.

To achieve this, we, temporary earth's off spring, so delicate, so stupid and so smart have at our disposition but a short life-span to observe our surroundings — with the help of scarce beacons stretched over a few thousand years only.

Until recently, we ignored the number of centuries, eras and periods that the planet has harboured us so far. We proceed by relying on two unique variables, time and space, that define the Cartesian plane of our lives.

My stay on earth is substantially minute, noticeably short and my comments are markedly insignificant. They do not break any sound barrier or force any dead end. Rationally it would be better for me not to disclose them. Affectively also. Indeed, what is not said will not ridicule anyone.

But my silence could be seen as incomprehension.

If on the other hand, I express my findings too eloquently, I will be assumed to be arrogant and my critics will fiercely look for cracks in my logic.

They will decapitate my chapters and remove paragraphs. My dislocated sentences will be just like the heterogeneous words of the local newspapers' necrology.

Easy job.

With care and humility I shall risk presenting those jigsaw pieces that I could not refrain from collecting. They have in my view the authority of contemplating a disease called fatigue from another perspective, as well as other diseases whose origins are too often ignored and whose treatment could lead to Baudelaire's words:

"My child, my sister,
Consider tenderness
To live there together
There, everything is but order and beauty,
Luxury, calm and sensuality."

Those precious clues scattered over centuries recall the tumultuous path of a category of intracellular micro-organisms, which have the potential of massive human destruction even though they seem perfectly tame most of the time.

My description does not include their hidden lives, or their future lives, but will be an attempt at scientific reflection of their striking exploits and some of their underhanded acts.

Our aggressors X, Y and Z will plead not guilty, just like we would do in the war free of armistice, called survival.

A nation of classification against another.

Because rickettsia and its close pathologic agents colonise our cytoplasm, we become the secret garden of these parasites. They set the stage and orchestrate our lives, from the network of our tissues through which they proceed masked.

CHAPTER 1:

GERMS' CIVILISATION
AROUND OUR CIVILISATION

"The truth is too simple,
one always must get there by the complicated."
—*George Sand*—

Dear Reader

You are a lawyer, a businessman, a builder, a sportsman, an actor, an artist, a pilot or a farmer and life goes well for you. Whoever you are, are you interested in germs? Because they are interested in you. They consider you the bridge between your life and theirs.

Germs will be with us as long as life exists.

In order to survive, nature takes from one part to give to another.

By instinct.

A shark devours a surfer with no more passion than fleas bite cats, boys eat broccoli and cocks mate with hens — or streptococcus infects tonsils. Pestilences just need fuel to cross the world.

They are fighting to subsist.

For every one that survives, a thousand die. Just like the tide of freshly-hatched turtles rushing off to the sea; how many reach adulthood?

We only realise their existence when they enter our lives. They display an invasive power and meet a resistant power. The change of equilibrium between these two powers produces oscillations between epidemic, attenuated and dormant forms of parasites throughout the history of species on each continent.

Seventy years ago, in 1933, the concept of 'attenuated forms of diseases' was described by Charles Nicolle as the survival of germs on earth that had lost their virulence due to the resistance force developed against them.

From this study on infectious diseases' destiny, it follows that every germ has many kinds of existence. First, each one has an individual life in the isolated body used for its survival, as each one of us needs a place to nest. Subsequently, reaching a multitude of individuals, the disease goes through a blazing epidemic phase. It is its golden age. And if this epidemic phase shines enough to change the destiny of a few civilisations, its glory will travel down the ages; this is the historical phase.

Making fun of time and space, the final word belongs to the ambiguous life. At each moment it will decide, and tolerate or reject, the association with live particles — a never-defined conclusion between life and death.

A banal acquaintance could turn into a nightmare if pH, temperature, magnetism or other physical phenomena get involved. A basic unicellular organism could change our destiny with the same power as the Big Bad Wolf on Little Red Riding Hood, when a multicellular one, complex and fascinating, lacks aggressive stratagems. Justice is absent even from the infinitesimal life.

In a constant declaration of war, our body must adapt or fight the elements around us. If we fail to adjust, we become a statistic in history, a dodo in the chapter of the disappeared species.

The virulence of the micro-organisms surrounding us could reoccur at any time after changes of circumstances. It will only take them a few mutations. The outbreak of epidemic diseases is often seen when a large concentration of people is agglomerated in cities, and where communication with other parts of the world is unruly. The process will become inevitable if, furthermore, military troops are moving backwards and forwards.

The circumstances that met in the Italy of the 6th century, when barbarian immigrants were occupying the land, were quite similar to what happens in today's Europe, where the social system is attractive and where armies are sent to other countries, such as Bosnia, the Middle East and Central Africa. This occurs daily on many contemporary continents.

Through all times, political migrations, caused by civil wars or international conflicts, will add to economic migrations. Also religions and fanatics will push millions on the road to disease.

To add here, the contribution of the growing tourism industry is an ideal recipe to achieve an outstanding growth medium. The environment selects those mutant forms most suitable to reproduce. Otherwise, the item will be discontinued.

"In the wild, species are beautiful because the male, the strongest, chases rivals away and enjoys the female." Antoine Rivarol, French writer, 1753-1801, noticed, foreseeing Darwin's Theory of Evolution. But first let us try to define similarities between power and beauty.

Pasteur also observed natural selection.

This explains the appearance and disappearance of contagious diseases through History, as wrote Charles Nicolle: " because infectious diseases have an historical life, just like any alive organism, they are born, grow and modify through ages" i.e. being infected and having nothing to show to the doctor and to yourself, or being infected and still appearing healthy. That was Charles Nicolle's paradox.

At the individual level, infectious diseases present in three different stages:

Hidden disease — where earth and insects are vectors

of virulent agents and where men are carriers of those same agents, but stay asymptomatic. The perfidious and secret breeding of germs takes place here. The epidemic proportions of a disease are reduced to small endemic pockets. This simulates its eradication, although the pathologic potential is there. At this stage, it only needs trauma, psychological stress, malnutrition, or harsh climatic conditions for the agent to explode into virulence. It is saprophytic by accident.

Acute disease — where man displays suddenly known signs of the infection. From saprophytic, the parasite becomes opportunistically pathogenic.

Chronic disease — where the carrier still has the germ of a previous infection more or less contained, for more or less time.

The factors producing the passage of a disease from a dormant form to an active one are numerous and intricate, and do not make sense to our logical thinking.

Signals are sent continuously in our blood. Our cells decode these messages and organise defence mechanisms all around our body, addressing different systems.

It is a star war. Our brain is ignorant of this fight, unless it goes wrong.

How to define the balance between health and illness? Our scientists spend a lot of time noting things going wrong, instead of trying to understand what is going right.

Microbes, their reservoirs, their hosts and their environment form an ecosystem. This is the most complex level of organisation in nature. Some of our intrusions inside this system, meaning well, could lead to the opposite.

A study done by Paul Giroud et al, published in the Bulletin de la Société de Pathologie Exotique in 1962, serves as a good example of the hazardous guess that can take place after introducing a chemical novelty into our almost unpredictable ecosystem. It demonstrated that most strains of toxoplasm are harmless to white rats, but that Toxoplasma gondii might cause a fatal disease if infected rats are treated with steroids. The author concludes: "These steroids might therefore constitute a hazard in children and pregnant women." Besides the fact that the restriction to children and women, pregnant above all, is unclear to my mind, this could find an unexpected application in our daily medicine.

It's very difficult to codify those ecosystem's laws into our world. Maybe some valuable indices could be revealed by using two complementary approaches. Firstly, the scientific mind progresses carefully from one deduction to the next, covering ground logically and sensibly in one planned direction. Secondly, the intuitive approach suddenly establishes unexpected links between two facts, leading to untaught concepts.

The strictness of a logical deduction is the essence of any scientific progress. However, without an imaginative inspiration, it will lose its vital boost.

Nicolle wrote: "Triggered by us or not, the spike

shoots up, unexpected, brutal, flashing. The moment before, everything was darkness, confusion, and torpor. Suddenly, everything becomes crystal clear, obvious. It is a revelation... This shock, this sudden lighting, this self-possession through a new fact, I am able to speak about. I have felt them. I have lived them. This jump forward, this conquest of the unknown of yesterday is an act, not of reasoning, but of imagination, intuition. It is an act limited to the artist and to the poet, a dream which seems a creation."

Today one would speak about the right and the left brain. The right hemisphere analyses, the left hemisphere realises. The same information could lead to a completely different conclusion, depending on to which side of the brain the word is given.

Some of us give more sway to the right brain, others listen more to the left. They are the intellectual and the physical, dreamers and builders. Some dreamers build, as do some builders dream. Because, at night, if everything goes well, the two brains communicate. The right receptor, after visiting the Collective Unconscious of Carl Jung, a kind of spiritual website for surfing the whole humanity, sends its mail to the left brain. The latter has the power to materialise the concepts sent by the former. The quality of communication between the two brain hemispheres determines the leap forward taken by Charles Nicolle, just like the ones of so many other geniuses, artists and musicians.

CHAPTER 2:

GHOSTS THROUGH GEOGRAPHY AND HISTORY IN MEDICINE

Oh this fever, do not assail me.
— Spell recited by the Egyptians to prevent the
entrance of disease-laden vapours — 1600 B.C. —
Breasted, 1930

Very often the medical world ignores the concept of parasitic virulence working in successive waves through history and geography. Consequently new names appear to define old diseases. What an epigram those medical books will be, in abbreviated editions, scattered with white pages after a remix of parasites, protozoas and other disguised ghosts.

In a common effort to avoid being swallowed up,

they play hide and seek through the centuries and regularly shake the human destiny. Some are losing, some are winning.

The ephemeral do not have the same pathological input, as do the enduring ones. Let us try to trace a few of them.

We could start with the fairly newborn Lyme disease. This disease was named after the town in Connecticut, where Borrelia burgdorferi was isolated in 1975, after a mysterious outbreak of arthritis near Lyme. The sixteenth edition of the Merck Manual, a professional handbook published on a non-profit basis as a service to the scientific community, taken amongst others, serves as an example. It speaks about a newly-discovered spirochete in the USA. No mention is made of its possible link with the recurrent Malgache fever, caused by the spirochete Borrelia duttoni — not in here, not in other medical indexes.

In 1911, Thézé described the first appearance of this spirochete, Borrelia duttoni, ignoring in a similar way the journals of the scientist Drury, dated from 1702 to 1720, and reporting the existence of the same disease, following the bite of the tick called 'ornithodorus moubata' in Central Africa.

Recurrent literally means 'running back on its tracks'. Also called recurrent fever, this illness causes deep fatigue, headaches, muscle and joint aches, all symptoms shared with rickettsial infection.

The Spirochete hispanicum was identified in the early 1900s in Spain. Charles Nicolle later tracked it in northern Africa. This condition is now known as Hispanico African fever and its symptoms are similar to those of Lyme disease.

Scheltz was working in the Belgian Congo in 1933 and reported the same recurrent fever, and (surprise) the presence of the same spirochete to blame.

After him, and again without knowledge of each other's discovery, in 1944, Palakov published proudly and, yes, with reason that the relapsing fever disabling patients in Cape Town was due to the same bug.

It also happened that Heisch was in Kenya in 1950 to claim the recognition of borreliosis as causing that never-ending fever (Bulletin de la Société de Pathologie Exotique — 1952).

Today, the diagnosis of this condition is arduous and based only on clinical findings. Laboratory testing is still in its early stages, although its corkscrew profile when seen through the microscope is not more enigmatic than its DNA structure.

A few pioneers have recommended antibiotherapy, while still arguing about the type and the length of the treatment.

More and more this infection is thought to be escorting other pathogenic agents carried by ticks (Burrascano). This is a logical consequence of the way ticks live in dirt and feed off wild animals, which become reservoirs of the disease.

Further, what of that other spirochete responsible for syphilis, presenting the same type of slow moving evolution in its host? How could we evaluate the number of its victims and the length of its reign?

What an ingenious ghost. It manages to enter the human body through genital or other mucosae. Then, at the point of looking revolting, it vanishes without leaving any trace — except an unexpected recovery.

One among others, that profits from the naïve and optimistic human mind to ensure prosperity before the enemy awakes.

Two months later, the prey suffers from headaches, sore throat, low-grade fever and a rash. Confusing brine of bacterial or viral infection that could give the change for rubella or chicken pox. These rashes disappear under the same magic wand. This is the secondary phase. A short period brings the ignorant patient to the latent phase and the final tragedy. The latent phase is a condition of well being, much welcome after these unexplained malaises.

Unfortunately the first two phases are extremely contagious.

The pale treponema then falls into a deep sleep. Sometimes even death will not wake it up. However, years later, insidiously, syphilitic gummas will form and wreck any tissue. Dementia and general paralysis are not the only symptoms.

Furthermore, syphilis is transmitted from the mother

to the foetus through the placenta. Abortion or perinatal death is a consequence of the infection. If still alive, the infant can be blind with foggy patches on the cornea, or deaf following involvement of the auditory nerve. His chipped teeth frighten little children and his nose looks like a cooking-pot's leg.

This merciless nightmare took and takes over many bodies regardless of their rank. Tsars, kings or their subjects are equally at risk. Therefore, Russia collapsed for more than half a century in chaos proportional to the size of the land and to the position of the gummas in the brain of Ivan the Terrible.

Before Alexander Flemming and the discovery of penicillin in 1928, syphilis was treated with laxatives and magic antidotes directed against the disease — treatment amazingly similar to the one in use today to cure Chronic Fatigue Syndrome (CFS). The fashion suggests colono-therapy, alternated with hydrotherapy and other detoxification regimes. In 1917, a law was passed in England: any non-qualified 'therapist' treating symptoms was committing a criminal offence.

In 1905, two German scientists discovered the pathogenic agent of syphilis. They called it Spirochaeta pallida, which was later to become Treponema pallidum.

The Wasserman test was discovered in 1906. In those days, chemists and doctors were looking for the perfect antiseptic to inject into the blood. The aim was to destroy the germs without affecting the tissues. The first 'systemic antiseptic' was discovered in 1910 and named '606' or 'magic ball'. The yellow powder, an arsenic derivative called salvarsan, proved to be toxic to the tissues and inefficient against the treponema. More research lead to an effective chemical: neo salvarsan. It was used during World War 1, when syphilis was at the height of its notoriety.

Today, in Africa, syphilis puts bread and butter on the table of the GP that is happy to inject a bottle of penicillin. At least he can treat the disease before notification to the health department, should anyone up there be really interested — unless he is prepared to spend time to achieve both tasks.

A direct application of this medical history would be an edict making syphilis testing compulsory for all, including the higher echelon of government, as prevention against some nationwide delays and setbacks.

Malta fever, first described as transmitted by goat's milk, is also a member of this swirl of the raving mad. Its first name comes from the Island of Malta, where it appeared early in the nineteenth century.

It is a remarkable disease considering its geographic distribution. It is found in the Middle East, Africa and all over Europe. Its rapid evolution is characteristic. Starting with fever, any organ may become involved and lead to severe complications, just as in tuberculosis, which it seems to copy.

27

Charles Nicolle, with his visionary mind called it "the disease of the future". Today, we find it attacking farmers, vets and cattle. It is called brucellosis.

The disease is contracted after eating or drinking the products of an infected animal or by direct contact through a cutaneous abrasion, by the conjunctiva or by inhaling contaminated dust. This calamity is found in different hosts, probably after appropriate mutations. The name varies and describes its habitat or its function: it is called Brucella melitensis when it inhabits sheep, Brucella suis when it infests pigs and Brucella abortus in cattle when infected cows abort, Brucella rangiferi when it attacks the Arctic caribou and Brucella canis in dogs.

The disease is still often misdiagnosed, and if by any chance treatment is applied, it is long and does not protect from frequent relapses.

Tuberculosis flourishes particularly well hand-in-hand with poverty. No continent has managed to eradicate it yet. Despite excellent knowledge of the disease, diagnosis, pathogenicity and widespread vaccine campaigns, there is no guarantee of being protected one hundred percent and anybody, rich or poor, may one day be visited.

Century after century, country after country, it invades insidiously the weak and malnourished or, in association with another pathological monster, throws their common target into eternity.

How do we recognise the real culprit in the historical

and geographical epic, or in medical terms, what is the cause of death? What exactly will be written on the death certificate reserved for the next statistics?

In the middle of these diseases going into the humanity conquest, there is still Leishmaniasis, described as Kala-Azar in India by two English bacteriologists, Leishman and Donovan.

That was 1903. The name of the disease was decided in that year, although the parasite had already been recognised by Cunningham in 1885. The disease induced high fever with black pigmentation of the skin. Kala Azar means 'high fever' in the Hindu language.

Beside Leishmania donovani, Charles Nicolle isolated, in 1908, Leishmania tropica, a disease in which the reservoir is the dog and which is transmitted to humans by a skin parasite. It was not uniformly distributed in the Tunis population when it attracted Nicolle's attention. Italians, living in poor areas, were the most infected. Then came the French. In third position were the Muslims. Strangely, the Israeli community did not develop the disease. It was therefore logical to think that those different groups presented a higher sensitivity to the disease, or deployed fewer defence mechanisms.

Listening to his intuition and not to his logic, Nicolle examined the different groups of sick people. If group one and two are sick, but differently, and if group three is clear of the disease, it means there is a factor common to the first two groups but distributed differently, and this factor is absent in the third group.

What could this factor be? Nicolle found it. It was the dog, the reservoir of the disease.

Of course, the French had dogs, but the Italians lived in shacks in a promiscuous environment. Muslims had dogs, but did not treat them as domestic animals. Israelis had practically no dogs.

In 1925, while travelling in Argentina, Nicolle once more isolated the American forest leishmania. It was called Leishmania brasiliens.

In 1937, cases of leishmania were isolated in France. L. chagasi is rife in Central America, specially Honduras. Let us quote also L. major, parasiting populations from Afghanistan to Africa, L. archibaldi in East Africa and others which are carrying the name of their invaded country: L. mexicana, L. venezuelensis or pifanoi, L. amazonensis, L. peruviana, and eventually L. panamensis.

We must emphasise the increasing amount of leishmaniasis as well as tuberculosis in patients suffering from AIDS, in whom immunity is collapsing following the reduction of Lymphocytes T CD4.

The treatment of leishmaniasis is as precarious and medieval as the name of the chemical: an antimony derivative.

One hundred years after its discovery, where is the research concerning leishmaniasis? Still the historical and geographical extent of the disease seems to be whispering an invitation to today's scientist. The difficulty lies in the fact that they are invited everywhere, these druids of a science as new as medicine.

In this medical trail also walks another virulent 'ugly' called toxoplasmosis. It equally does not suffer from apoplexy.

Nicolle first described toxoplasmosis in 1907, as being part of the leishmaniasis species. He called it Leishmania gundii, after he isolated it from the Ctenodactylus gundi, a small rodent found in the area surrounding Tunis.

Later on, because the parasite did not grow in the same medium as leishmania, it was reclassified. Due to technical improvements, the germ appeared clearly as a crescent that gave it its new name: Toxoplasma gondii from the Greek toxon meaning 'bow'.

This infection can present as an acquired or congenital form, acute or chronic, generalised or localised. In the brain, heart, skin, eyes, glands. Anywhere its evolution can be slow, in the shelter of a dark cyst. It can cause abortion or severe visual impairment in the newborn.

Today this serious disease is widespread and, despite intensive researches following its fortuitous discovery, the treatment is difficult, relapses are frequent and very often the diagnosis is missed. As a typical scrounger, it keeps a place of honour in the gloomy cortege following AIDS.

Another historical ghost is personified by the bubonic plague, a disease caused by Yersinia pestis, transmitted to humans all over the world by the flea of the rat.

The rat, again, with his face resembling an answer to any epidemiological enigma.

One can easily imagine a port in the south of England. Let us set it up in the early fourteenth century; fog, steaming quays, songs and screams of drunken sailors going through the night. One can hear the screech of the hull slowly pitching in the lapping water, and from this magnificent sailboat, surface ropes go to mooring posts. She comes back from a long journey in the Middle East. The untidy deck indicates the exhaustion of the crew and the relief when they drop anchor. Then, looking harder, one could perceive a movement on a rope and recognise the shadow of a rat, a stowaway coming from the East.

This rat is a carrier of death. The Black Death, which will change history.

In the trail of this awkward-gaited and ignorant rat, humanity will find disappearances, insanity, misery, devastation and an unbelievable emptiness. Deserted houses, smouldering towns, lonely survivors wandering aimlessly, children suckling the breast of a dead mother, ghost ships throwing overboard decomposed passengers before sinking on the rocks...

Is it feasible to see today the same political, socio-economic and cultural turmoil in and around the pit caused by AIDS? Are we at the dawn of an unprecedented continental or even world concussion?

Our planet so often criticised will be cleared of human life. How fortunate. No more fight about the ozone layer. No more of the same old refrain about pollution, black tides and their cortege of oily seals. No more technical hazards leading to death, no more nuclear catastrophe. No more overpopulation. No population anymore. We are not here to disturb nature.

Next one.

"Who inhabited this place before me?" asks the walking, newly-skinned chameleon. How many times will it have to clean its chromosomal dusts before having access to the next clone? How many cosmic radiations is it supposed to go through before reaching the next Big Bang?

No need to be a palm reader to explain the logic of this utopia. No need to be a chemist to explain alchemy.

Need of the present to explain the future?

Plague will always be a frightening subject. It stayed in Europe and in Asia during centuries in an endemic stage. The first pandemic was reported in the sixth century after Christ, with an estimated few million deaths.

The second pandemic happened in the fourteenth century and was described as the Black Plague after the colour of the vanishing cyanotic patients. Fifty million people died, equivalent of fifty percent of the general population in those days.

During the centuries, in Africa and in Europe, one epidemic followed the other. The last pandemic started in China in 1894, and spread across the world to reach the United States in 1900. Today wild rodents are carriers on every continent, except perhaps Australia. The human disease persists in some endemic pockets, in some countries of Asia, Africa and South America.

Dyonisius described it in the third century before Christ.

Albert Camus in 1947, in his brilliant book, The Plague, traced the epidemic, which raged in Oran, Algeria. He starts: "On the morning of the 16th April 1940, Dr Bernard Rieux, coming out of his surgery, nearly tripped over a rat."

The analogy of the epidemic with the misery of war is obvious, and the scientific description of the infection is seriously respected. This allegoric work finishes with these words: "Let us listen, indeed. To the joyous shouts coming from town, Rieux remembered that this joy was always threatened. For he knew what this happy crowd ignored, and what one could get from a book, that the plague bacillus never died or disappeared, but that it can sleep for dozens of years, in furniture and fabric, that it will wait patiently in rooms, cellars, trunks, handkerchiefs and paper, and maybe the day will come for the misfortune of man; the plague will awaken its rats and send them to die in a happy city."

In this grim scenario yellow fever also features.

The yellow fever 'from town' is transmitted through the bite of a mosquito, carrying the poetic name of Aedes aegypti, which had been infected while biting a contaminated patient two weeks previously.

The yellow fever 'from the jungle' is transmitted through a small forest mosquito. The mystery of this infection starts with an orgy spent on wild primates. For the two forms, treatment is only symptomatic and sadly inefficient.

Trypanosomiases are classified into two groups of surly protozoas.

The first group consists of Chagas disease. The pathogenic agent is Trypanosoma cruzi. Its name comes from Carlos Chagas, a Brazilian who in 1909 observed the parasite in the intestine of the 'reduve', a loathsome insect which transmits the disease while stuffing itself with blood — its only activity. The disease exhibits cutaneous, cardiac, digestive and neurological symptoms. It chastises those countries from Central to South America, where it follows in the tracks of AIDS. The possibility of healing is mentioned in the treatment.

Sleeping sickness represents the second group. Trypanosoma brucei gambiense is transmitted by hanging onto the proboscis of the tsetse fly. This fly moves very little, lives in some areas of Africa and is a glutton, feeding every single day. Trypanosoma brucei rhodesiense is an acute form of the sleeping sickness.

In 1857, Livingstone mentioned the relationship between the tsetse fly bite and a state of drowsiness. But it was only in 1902 that Castellani described the parasite in Uganda.

This disease expresses with a sudden laziness, the face of a greedy guinea pig and the neck of an ostrich, which seems to have swallowed a few jewels to testify to the passage of tourists. This is caused by cervical gland hypertrophy. It was a criteria used by the slave drivers in the eighteenth century to select slaves in their trade with the West Indies.

This protozoa takes up residence preferably in humans or in dogs, but also in camels, pigs, cows, goats and sheep.

In 1912, Laveran wrote about them in a never-ending book with more than one thousand pages. Trypanosomes organelles mitochondria live just like bacteria in the cytoplasm, and my father suggested the possibility that pathogenic bacteria or virus could be carried inside Protozoa.

It is principally an African disease, found in endemic and epidemic forms. Its victims are thus far a medical novelty. It is found from Central Africa to the Zimbabwean borders, and in Latin America. My father managed to isolate it from the blood of bats that were haunting our attic in Antwerp.

When I suspect the disease in one of my patients, it is impossible to find a laboratory in Africa that practices the research of either its antibodies or its antigens.

The treatment requires arsenic. But often the infection is fatal.

And what malicious gossip to tell about malaria what everybody does not already know?

You do not find it only in tropical areas.

It is on the run in our history books, from the Ancient Egypt of 1550 B.C., and on every continent, from various papyri, swamp vapours and marshes. Our spiritual father Hippocrates knew perfectly the cycle of fevers it displays.

We do not try to eradicate it but only to control it. Once in your system, you will never be free of it. It signs its endemic condition by almost doubling the volume of the spleen, an organ situated close to the left kidney. Because, if malaria does not become obvious, it will settle in the reticulo-endothelial system, where it starts a long stimulation causing the spleen to dilate.

Malaria means in Italian 'filthy air', and indeed air is lousy in the swamps around Rome, which in Latin translate as 'palus' or 'marsh-fever'.

The vector of this fever is an anopheles, a mosquito that haunts those marshes and stays permanently in a curtsey position, even while biting you.

Quinine is an extract of the bark of the Cincocha tree, named after the princess who chewed it to alleviate her bout of fever. It was the only remedy used from 1679 till

1835. Vitelleschi, General of the Jesuits, discovered it in Peru in 1638. That miraculous medicine was then introduced in Europe by Talbot — an English warrior who was involved in the Hundred Year War — in powder form, called 'Jesuit powder' or 'English powder'. As soon as its composition was known publicly, it became fashionable to consume it as tea or coffee, because of its relaxing and aphrodisiac properties.

Then came DDT, to fight the anopheles. Its untimely use created, in no time, resistance from the mosquito. A little later, genetic changes arose in the flora touched by this chemical. Furthermore, its powerful impact affects targets and non-targets without differentiation.

The shortage in the production of quinine soon created a new problem, and researchers again started to try to find new methods of fighting malaria — single products or combined therapy. Nevertheless, quinine remains the best seller, except in cases of resistance.

Malaria remains a fierce killer of humankind. It kills between one and three million people every year – half a holocaust per annum.

But, to keep its status as queen of its empire, it has to cope with a setback compared with other diseases of the same calibre; instead of ignoring its existence, people work towards its eradication.

Exanthematic typhus is probably the champion of our scourges.

This giant killer counts to its credit a series of

carnage, and seems to adapt silently to any tissue, so long as it may from time to time cruise the vascular system.

This type of invasion allows this germ to carry an impressive number of pathological masks. The best investigator would lose his way.

Because of its exceptional survival possibilities, it survives for a long time in nearly any type of atmospheric condition. Its only need is to be contained in a certain type of reservoir or parasite, a temporary guest-house. This characteristic makes it indestructible.

Before the big leap of Charles Nicolle, very little was known about it. Its name originates from the two main symptoms: typhus, which means a state of stupor, and exanthema, which translates as skin rash.

The early stage of the infection may be slow or acute. First, it appears like a severe bout of flu. Fever develops quickly with shivers, depression, headaches and muscle pain in the limbs. A rash appears on day five, starting first on the shoulders and trunk, then spreading to the extremities. A typical sign is its presence on palms and soles. We have to look there to establish the diagnosis. These signs, associated with severe headaches, are strongly indicative of typhus, and should lead immediately to beneficial treatment without waiting for lengthy biological confirmation.

Typhus was always thought to be a unique and remarkable disease, different from other febrile infections. After studying the disease in the early twentieth century, we know that typhus is one of the most significant rickettsial infections.

During antiquity and the Middle Ages, it was mistaken for the plague. Thucydides describes a 'plague' in his 'Peloponnesian's war', which is according to the historian more likely to be a typhus. In Athens, fleas were following the move to town of peasants and their goats escaping the Lacedemonians, and devoured Socrates and his disciples. As Gerald Messadie writes in his exciting novel, *Madame Socrate*, "Three people were suffering from a particular illness. Gripped by a high fever, a severe laryngeal and ocular inflammation, then intractable diarrhoea, their skin was spotted by red dots and their general condition having deteriorated, their heart, or their kidneys, or their brain collapsed. After those three, eleven more citizens from the same area died. The frightening sight was the gangrene spreading to the extremities. Limbs were becoming purple then black and decomposed with an unbearable stink on those bodies where the heart was still beating. Those poor souls were witnessing their own decay and the worms crawling in their wounds. Death was deliverance. Lacedemonian spies were accused of poisoning wells. Then another one hundred and twenty people perished in the same conditions..."

Doctors were dying; undertakers and their paid mourners were dying; everyone was talking only about this, until the talking also had to stop.

Appalling epidemic.

One day you have everything, a bright mind, a handsome body, prosperity. The following day nothing is left, nor decency, nor law.

After the epidemic is gone, the memory of it equally disappears.

According to Zinsser, typhus started its political career in 1528, when Lautrec was commanding the French troops at the siege of Naples. Typhus hit the General. He died followed by the majority of his army. After the death of thirty thousand men, the battle ended.

One will find it again during the Hundred Years War.

Later it devastated the revolutionary troops and the Emperor's army during the 1877 war between the Turks and the Russians.

In Russia, again the same ghost murdered, without visible problem, three million people and weakened a further twenty-five million, according to Tarassewitch, then a scientist in Moscow. It was during World War I and between 1917 and 1923.

Following this huge number of victims, research on typhus grew rapidly, thanks to the work of Zinsser made easier by the research of Nicolle who was leading his investigation since 1903 in Djouggar, a native prison in the south of Tunis where an endemic of typhus was rife.

For Charles Nicolle, typhus was soon a priority among all the questions arising from the African continent. "It is the most important, the most unexplored."

41

What to do, to restore the energy needed to study these germs? How to wake up the deaf, the blind, and here, now, immediately on this planet I still belong to? The anorexia of all those silent years, where one can only find a few snatches in publications about rickettsiae. A few light and sporadic words written carefully, so as not to wake up the historic patriarch.

It is striking.

This subject is not insignificant. It is not old fashioned. Its empire is strong, opposed to our stillness. If anything could silence me on the spot, it is the patient and polite attitude that some people take while they wait for me to finish my words about rickettsiae.

At a pinch, those same people would accept opening the chapter on chlamydias, or quibbling about mycoplasma, as it was a new discovery in the United States.

In the scientific world, no one speaks about rickettsiae. Consequently, they do not exist any more. Let's call the first statement A, and the second B. A is correct. A implies B. Therefore B is also correct.

In other words, if it is true that I take my umbrella as soon as it rains, the fact of taking my umbrella will not make it rain.

The forgery in this syllogism is in the lack of research before exposing the affirmation.

How important is this discrimination? A long absenteeism often ennobles the dear departed when it reappears, but could also stick it in oblivion.

This is where our knowledge about rickettsiae fails.

They are not mentioned on the pathologist request form, or only in small print in the shadow of the word 'Weil Felix'. The Micro-agglutination test of Giroud, the pioneer of rickettsial serology, is forgotten. Today's techniques in modern laboratories are obviously more advanced, compared with that manual, slow and costly test.

Is it sufficient reason to forget the disease?

Perhaps it is time to replace the test, or to modernise it, and certainly, if nothing else, to provide us with new antigens in the meanwhile.

Otherwise, the diagnosis, the treatment and the recovery of people suffering from chronic rickettsial infection might have to be interrupted due the lack of antigens available to perform the test.

Unfortunately, today's research is directed more towards genetic engineering and trying to auction more spectacular subjects, leaving the rickettsiae of the past in limbo. While decrypting mistakes responsible for hereditary diseases or isolating pieces of DNA, we will not meet the immunological eccentricities generated by contact with rickettsia. Still people suffer the disease all around the globe — sometimes with the uncertain privilege of dying quickly from it…

Here again, a new typhus epidemic. We are in 1912, in the middle of a Balkan war. And once more, at the end of the twentieth century, in the same place, emerges another mysterious Balkan's syndrome, with fatigue as the main symptom. Soldiers that the United Nations sent to Bosnia and Kosovo are back home today and are still suffering from ... a mixture of typhus and rickettsial-like diseases.

In Kuwait, in 1978, the epidemic coincided with a period of high density of rats and flies in town. Typhus threw a party.

Him, taking part in the disaster in 1991, where his close relatives have been isolated, during the Gulf war?

Close to the exanthematic typhus, there are still other strains.

We will only mention here the Rickettsia mooseri, transmitted by rats using fleas to penetrate humans. It is less lethal than epidemic typhus, but is an invasive disease, capable of organ destruction, alike the kidney and the heart of Charles Nicolle. Also known as endemic typhus, the murine disease can develop in epidemic form and kill as efficiently as the old war typhus. Identified in 1950 by J-B Jadin as being the agent of Congo red fever, it spreads from the equator to South Africa.

Is there also a typhus trick behind the recent powerful reappearance of CFS, the famous chronic fatigue syndrome? This disease is also called ME for myalgic encephalomyelitis, or Yuppie flu to describe the type of people who are susceptible to it.

This worldwide illness is not new. In the nineteenth century the neurologist George Beard from New York gave it its first popular name: neurasthenia. In the middle of the twentieth century, neuromyasthenia came along to emphasise the muscular weakness found in this condition.

Could CFS be a new name, not only for neurasthenia or neuromyasthenia or ME and Yuppie flu, but also for rickettsial-like diseases?

I said 'rickettsial-like' because this parasite is able to undergo any kind of face-lift to save its life, such as to get a membrane around itself, or lose a few enzymes, and change shape and size.

It happened after all in the experiments of Giroud to the extent of injecting a strain of Rickettsia mooseri into rats and, according to the host metabolic activity or the substrate on which they grow, getting a strain of Rickettsia conori out there, which was not found previously. Paul Giroud confirmed this phenomenon in a second experiment, where he passed a conori strain from a mouse's lung to an egg's membrane; it grew and acquired the characteristics of a mooseri. Names of different species of rickettsiae found around the globe could number 100. Some of them are probably identical.

Indeed CFS was first reported in Incline Village, Nevada, in 1984, where it developed in epidemic proportions. Rocky Mountain Spotted Fever is caused by a rickettsia and originated from the same place in 1916. In fact, CFS and rickettsial infections share the same symptoms.

Rickettsia senetsui is the pathogenic agent of some types of glandular fever, all sharing the same symptoms as infectious mononucleosis. Could simple confusion between the two diseases indicate that the Epstein Barr virus, so often incriminated, is a cause of chronic fatigue?

Without a doubt, CFS patients, after being diagnosed as suffering from a rickettsial-like disease, will respond positively to anti-rickettsial treatment.

The Iceland outbreaks in 1886 and 1888, called Iceland disease, were also an epidemic neuromyasthenia. Nurses and ancillary institutional personnel were the most attacked. The symptoms involved nervous, muscular and reticulo-endothelial systems. Fatigue was the headline. Fever and lymphadenopathy were testifying to an infective aetiology.

Another reason for suggesting an association between CFS and chronic infection can be found in the link between Florence Nightingale and CFS. The reality that she was working, surrounded by lice, fleas and ticks, treating soldiers with wounds and with epidemic typhus during the Crimean war, could be a logical explanation as to why she was terribly tired during the last two decades of her life.

On the other hand, the lymphocyte population in the peripheral blood of different groups of CFS patients has been the subject of many studies. The results show similar changes. The study conducted in sheep experimentally infected with the causative agent of tick-born fever, show the same changes as those noted in the lymphocyte studies of patients suffering from Q fever endocarditis. We should mention here that Q fever is still generally classified as a rickettsial disease caused by Coxiella burnetti.

Should the enquiry continue, or do we prefer to keep untouched the fairytale that CFS already represents?

The epidemic forms of rickettsiae were described by Zinsser in his classic book Rats, Lice and History (Annals New York Academy of Sciences, 1990, ref) in which he contends that soldiers have rarely won wars. Typhus and other infectious diseases have decided the outcome of more military campaigns than Caesar in the Gallic conquest, Hannibal, when he crossed the Alps on his elephant's back, during the second Punic war, Napoleon in his Russian campaign, and all generals in history. Depending on the outcome for each warring faction, either the epidemics were blamed for defeat, or the generals were credited with victory.

The same typhus epidemic developed in the Nazi concentration camps.

So, typhus not only fluctuates with seasons, but also appears to be associated with stress, cold and malnutrition.

It is presently believed that following on from these historical memories, there are forms less virulent, evolving slowly, but able to induce vascular and neurological pathologies (Clinique de la Conférence du

Parc- Au sujet des maladies rickettsiennes, Annales de la société belge de médecine tropicale, 1962 volume 3).

Are you still there?

Did you follow me in that labyrinth packed with disgusting creatures? My intention was not to lose you, by dropping them as breadcrumbs instead of stones, nor to put you to sleep, counting germs instead of sheep, but to bring you face to face with the obvious, so that it can hurt you, as much as it hurts me.

Do not worry if you are bored to death, or depressed, or feeling exhausted after reading that endless number of diseases. Reading about them is about the only safe way to come close to them without catching them, but would you agree with me that I have just written a convincing essay on the sentence of Doctor Knock of Jules Romain: " All well men have a sickness waiting to happen"?

Writing this complaint too long and too dark on the Wailing Epidemiological Wall is not only a prose essay. Nor a beat to track pathological discoveries through the centuries.

Before everything, it is a calculated attempt to unveil good news, as numerous and as powerful as the bad news. It is called diagnosis, treatment and prevention.

I put on paper those shocking stories everybody wants to ignore, in a persistent and laughable hope that they will be read. Those horror masks drag on, unabated, thanks to our ignorance; espionage is a strategy capable of conquering many territories. Furthermore, against those scourges, there is a recipe. It will put you back on your feet, in good condition to continue your walk on this earth, the only one surely promised, which is our universe.

And if the recipe does not yet exist, it is time for discovery, because the main interest in your disease's story lies in its solution.

CHAPTER 3:

MY BACKGROUND

"About so many novelties I am not curious.
It pleasures me to imitate the train of my ancestors."
Pierre de Ronsard.

My father was from Lustin, a small village close to Namur, in the south of Belgium, where the river Meuse runs between cliffs and hills covered with apple trees, sheep and beehives. The perfume of this honey is as delicious to the sense of smell as the countryside is beautiful to the eye. This is why my father used to compare any striking scenery which he came across on his multiple voyages with these humble words: "It is nearly as beautiful as Lustin."

As a child he had three passions, which were canaries, cats and chess. Canary breeding was a laborious job. His schoolmasters were complaining, not considering the genetic knowledge he aquired that way.

Another demanding task was the love he lavished on his cats. He would even forgive them their hunter instinct and its interference with his first devotion. The rest of his time was spent with his beloved brother playing chess. One day, the turn of the game infuriated him so much that, armed with a chair, my father opened the skull of his brother.

The time spent as a medical student in Namur was devoted to never-ending card-playing sessions, specifically 'le couillon' and other student celebrations. His famous student toque that was supposed to contain beer at each festivity is still here as testimony to those crazy days.

After completing his specialisation in Medical Microbiology in Louvain, Belgium, he started his research at the Pasteur Institute in Tunis, with Charles Nicolle, winner of the Nobel Prize for Medicine in 1936.

During that time, a friendship grew between master and student, as witnessed by the correspondence they kept afterwards, discussing their ideas and their work.

My father was then commissioned by the Royal Institute of Belgium to study the blood groups and other anthropologic parameters of the legendary Pygmy tribes living in the luxuriant forests of Ituri, Congo.

They were, my father wrote, "primitive and millenary beings, still belonging to the dark ages, as if they could be ancestors of other men ".

The pygmies are individuals, who appear to be content with their fate, perfectly adapted and suited to the most abundant of environments. Authentic pygmies survive by harvesting wild honey and poaching in their equatorial forest. The Ruwenzori mountains, called 'Hills of the Moon', and the equatorial plains through which flows the immense Congo River, are all subject to these weather conditions.

To live as they do, it is imperative that their environment is preserved.

The virgin forest provides them with this inextricable aspect where the vegetation is nourished by the humus formed as the dead leaves accumulate and rot on the forest floor. This process has been occurring systematically for centuries and there is no reason for it to stop yet. In these circumstances the vegetation is able to develop in its own way and interminably. From this fertile earth, trees fight their way to the light and rise through lianas so thick than Jane would have no chance of tracking her Tarzan.

They grow in height and width for as long as the unbridled elements allow them to. They then hinder the forest floor and render the dense foliage more impenetrable.

Of small size, the pygmy has a joyous nature and the present moment is the sole object of his thoughts. Therefore, both his joys and sorrows are short-lived.

The average size of the adult pygmy man is approximately 1,4 metres, and that of the woman is approximately 1,3 metres. They adorn themselves with strips of bark attained from the trees they have cut down.

The pygmy's entire life is oriented towards his hunting. Randomly, they establish camps where they will generally stay for a few days. At night, they gather around a fireplace to quietly discuss events, while smoking marijuana.

The pygmy will never leave his bow and arrows unattended, even when dancing. He makes use of fatal poison, originating from plants or animals.

Pygmies hunt in small groups. After storing their pipes in a tree trunk, they throw themselves into the pursuit of antelope, bush pig, or even large game, buffalo or elephant. They are able to detect the mere spoor and to hear the faintest sound. They climb and swing about in the tree branches, as agile as monkeys.

Their sharp weapons enable them to slash through an elephant's tendons, or to pierce its abdomen. Once the animal is wounded, its trunk is slit, or a lance is planted into the rectum to provoke a lethal haemorrhage.

The death of the beautiful animal happens with an infernal crash of falling trees, and fills your orifices with a red and adhesive dust. This avalanche is followed by an unimaginable orgy, inside the body of the victim, from whence come songs of victory and muffled cries of joy. The event is celebrated with great gulps of palm spirit.

The dull grey skin of the elephant transformes itself

little by little into a huge tent. This anachronic canopy deflates slowly as the elephant is eaten from the inside, a hunt trophy lit by primitive torches, flapping to the rhythm of the warrior's dances. They prolong their enjoyment until dawn and crawl out of the carcass replete, discoloured with blood and staggering, blinded by the morning sun.

The Ruwenzori mountains are forever in the mist, which enhances the disturbing atmosphere of this immeasurable sacrifice.

No spectator is invited.

If the pygmy is in danger of extinction, it is not because of his lack of courage or intelligence, but because of his physical anatomy that does not allow him to combat intruders physically more able in this ancient conflict involving two clashing nations.

After his colourful stay with the Pygmies, my father decided to pursue his work in Rwanda and Urundi, where I was born, number 6 out of a family of 7. He worked there and in Johannesburg, in collaboration with the late Professor James Gear of the South African Institute for Medical Research.

My childhood memories are both enchanting and horrific.

Images from a wonderland; like those of vaporous clouds exhaled from trunks becoming steam baths in the early morning moisture; like those of the mountain sketched in grey and white to welcome a few gorillas in the mist; mingled with terrifying war scenes between the Hutu and the Tutsi tribes.

Memories of elephant calves, which had been entrusted to my mother as local poachers had slaughtered their herds. I did not stop to wonder about the rapidity with which the orphaned calf drained his bucket of milk – much faster than the most powerful vacuum cleaner advertised on television.

The story of the leopard cub, which grew too big for our cat's safety and had to be placed in the zoo in Antwerp.

The scream of Joseph, the Chimpanzee in love with my mother, when he had to leave her to go back to his cage.

My father's lab and the goose flesh that sprayed over me when I crossed from the cold room to the one left at ambient temperature.

I often did not attend school.

Tribal struggle. Pictures of women and children, stumbling on their legs amputated at the knee, in a pool of their own blood to meet their death. The vengeance of one on an other.

Images of the sunrise, smells of the damp forest, colour of the earth red-orange of laterite, crocodiles, the diligent eye half closed in the river where we were floating in a dugout made of ebony, or formosa wood.

The rough lulled voice of our guides, singing a litany of what they were seeing, or what they were feeling – hunger, thirst, tiredness, wellbeing which they repeated unflaggingly, day after day, century after century.

Slithering snakes, exploded in sparkles when they would cross sunrays.

The powerful double bass of the nearby roaring lions.

The multicoloured birds with shrill, harmonious or aggressive song.

A tame barn owl, which would nestle on my shoulder at a whistle-blow, and who died, burned alive in the shed where she roosted. Innocent victim of black magic prophesy?

A small monkey named Jacquot that stayed in the orange tree in front of my window and fondled my hair with his small grimy fingers, as a mother grooming her child. I tried to say as quite as possible to facilitate his work. Not to hurt him. I did not know that these stereotyped gestures were part of the genetic memory of this species.

Terrifying thunderstorms, magnificent yet destructive, that sent me huddling under the dining-room table. Doors were banging, the first rain drops splashed the floor vigorously, electricity had left the lampposts and bounced freely in the ozone's smell, the lightening flashes were tearing the sky in giant zig-zags, the trees were uprooted and somewhere blood must have spurted out.

It was the end of the world. Since then, I never managed to be stormproof.

Flocks of African grey parrots, always accompanied by a raucous uproar, as well as a very peculiar odour, messengers of chlamydias.

The cruelty that the native Africans employed among themselves to maintain order, an example being the case of little Isidore, who had stolen beans and was punished accordingly. His hands were plunged in water still boiling.

I found again in South Africa those radical customs. For example, my domestic helper's ring finger was amputated. She had been stealing since childhood, and one morning as a lesson her grandmother chopped off the finger on the kitchen table. It is easy to understand the ineffictiveness of this barbaric technique, although so widely spread on the continent where I live.

The delicious perfume of roses that irrigated my nostrils and my skin damp after the rain.

A country violent and primitive, which stimulates the creativity in plenty.

A legendary nation where paradoxes are immense.

A wild and untamed land, burning with life, love and death, like a beautiful human pray.

In 1956, my father was nominated Professor of Protozoology and Haematology at the Institute of Tropical Diseases in Antwerp, Belgium, where we all went to live.

It was a coming back to civilisation.

I, therefore, entered European city life for the first time, other than for holidays.

The large and beautiful house in Antwerp was

charming, but I felt suffocated by the surrounding city.

The school I was to attend was a real nightmare. Not only was the spoken language, Flemish, which was totally unknown to me, but students were made to walk in rows and wear uniforms with a little hat similar to the ones of Napoleon's hussars. The school was also packed with stairs, which I did not know how to use. On my arrival and to the best of my knowledge, I attempted to climb the first flight of stairs on all fours. I felt that this achievement was crowned with shame, which started my bladder, and an even greater accident occurred before the collective and disjointed laughs of the other pupils. Here the origin of my second phobia, the stairs.

Little by little, I came to grips with this sad and grey country, where nothing was really familiar to me, and where everything appeared to me too organised amidst the filth and the boredom.

I was moved to another school. What an improvement this 'Lycée du Sacré Coeur' was, running for only a privileged few.

But besides this, I rebelled against my lost liberty and became the most conscientious of naughty pupils, organising protests worthy of the greatest vaudeville. At the top of the stairs coming down to the dining room, I was eavesdropping on the telephonic arguments between my parents, always lenient with their infant terrible, and the Mother Superior of the Sacre Coeur de Jesus, to whom I nearly gave a nervous breakdown.

My Wednesday afternoons were too often passed in detention, explaining Latin and Greek to boarders, who needed extra coaching. I particularly remember a pretty redhead, with luxuriant, curly hair and bouncing breasts. She suffered terribly from heavy periods and used to fill my ears with descriptions of her symptoms, like a prelude to my gynaecology course.

Altough some parts of Andromaque in the Euripide's version captivated me, for example this passage where she speaks about a man caressing her body as softly as a giant white soap, I would have far preferred Willy Kreitz's company, even if his tea was bitter.

Willy Kreitz was the director of the Fine Art Academy of Antwerp. Attending the same Rotary Club as my father, a friendship united them.

My father spoke to him about my determined and fanatical way of sketching everyone. Mr Kreitz kindly offered to teach me drawing every Wednesday afternoon. Some days and hours should not depend on any coincidence.

With joy, I managed to run simultaneously my dunce's fantasies and my academic schoolwork. Here it is necessary for me to render thanks to my good luck that has no common point with fortuity. Our teachers were the most cultivated and the French, Latin, Greek and Maths lessons were of the highest standard. Even by saving intellectual energy, it was difficult to be dumped.

My father also worked for many months in the

United States, at the Pasteur Institute in Paris, in Poland, in Greece and in Egypt.

During this time of his career, he travelled worldwide and accomplished 70 scientific trips. My mother often accompanied him and sometimes I was allowed to join them.

His enthusiasm and vitality were contagious.

He published about 500 scientific articles, mostly in French.

He was President or Member of more than 16 Scientific European Societies in Paris, Brussels, London, Athens, Moscow and Madrid. He was also a member of the Society of Protozoologists of the United States.

He was an authority on rickettsioses and neo-rickettsioses, on malaria, trypanosomiases, toxoplasmosis, leishmaniosis, leprosy and amoeba. Amongst these, one species of amoeba, Naegleria Jadini, was named after him. This was subject to the realisation of a movie shot in his laboratory, which suddenly was transformed into a Hollywood atmosphere. He had through this occasion the privilege to meet Antoine Derreumaux, specialist in pool system, which soon became a family's friend. It was to study those amoebaes that my father used his international contacts to gather samples of water from all over the world, including some mineral water so precious to the French people. Occasionally, he would isolate an amoeba, and his conclusion at an important conference in Antwerp in 1973 was noted: " From this day forward, I will recommend you to drink wine." Académie royale des sciences d'outre-mer 2000.

Many prizes honoured him.

On two occasions, in 1935 and 1938, he became laureat of the annual competition of the Royal Institut of the Belgium colonies. In 1946, he received the Broden Prize, of the Belgium Society of Tropical Diseases. In 1962, it was the Wertrems Prize, of the Royal Academy of Belgium. Then, in 1965, the E. Marchoux Prize was given to him by the Medical Academy of Paris.

He was nominated 'Grand Officier de l'Ordre de Leopold' and 'Grand Officier de l'Ordre de la Couronne'.

At the age of 91, he received his last prize for his research on rickettsial diseases and for the Microagglutination test. This was the Brumpt prize in 1997.

His colleagues were his friends and often they would gather for informal congresses in our home, first in the Belgian Congo, then in Antwerp or in the Castle of Arbre, our family holiday home near Namur.

Paul Giroud, Professor at the Pasteur Institute in Paris, developed the first vaccine against exanthematic typhus as well as the Micro-agglutination test for rickettsial diseases. Fifty years ago, he isolated Chlamydia trachomatis as the agent for Trachoma, which is the main cause of blindness in temperate and warm climates. He was a very intimate friend of the whole family and especially me. He used to call me 'la Parisienne', I was charmed by his humour, and his clear understanding that could present any complicated thought simply. When I can find good honey, I love to mix it with butter on a piece of toast and I remember hearing his beautiful voice, asking my mother for permission to indulge himself in this 'little filth'.

Paul Le Gag collaborated with my father in the campaign against the yellow fever epidemic in Central Africa, and initiated successful antibiotherapy for multiple sclerosis and similar conditions. The therapy I use for my fatigued patients is a direct result of his treatment. His publications, read in our days, have more the look of a prediction than of an outdated paper.

Maurice Mathis, famous entomologist, tick lover, and author of a wonderful book on bee's behaviour, was another friend of my father. He would never leave his ticks and lice behind, or maybe it was only lice? He also would never travel without his bees, and, when he did visit us, there was to be, sooner rather than later and without fail, a shortage of our concentrated fruit juice, that was diverted to keep the optimal activity in the beehive.

Pierre Vassiliadis, a very handsome man from Athens, who used to speak loudly with a rugged Greek accent, was a brilliant associate and friend, Director of the Hellenic Pasteur Institute.

There was also Professor Rud Geigy, from Basel, in

Switzerland. His letters were easily recognised in the post, marked with a pretty little wild boar, and he had a variety of dogs, which would not bark. Not that it was necessary because he was living in Switzerland, a country where quietness, infrastructure and safety is mastered, so that there is no need or advantage for a dog to bark.

Other friends were Professor Percy Cyril Garnham from the University of London, eminent protozoologist, who still wrote to me in 1991 when I started my treatment of chronic fatigued or rickettsial patients.

Robert Deschiens, director of the Société de Pathologie Exotique of the Pasteur Institut of Paris, was a real French gentleman who invited my sister and me to his holiday's apartment in Nice. He used to spoil us enormously in the best boutiques, the finest restaurants, looking for the best swimming pools with the highest diving-boards and the most succulent ice creams.

There was also Keith Vickerman, the specialist in trypanosomiases from Glasgow and Ben Rachid, from the Pasteur Institute of Tunis, who used to gather at the same 'café des nattes', in Sidi Bou-Saïd. Das, the specialist in amoeba, from India, Corliss from America, Cerva from Czechoslovakia, the Italians of Pavia University, Elio Rondanelli, Gan Pierro Carrosi and Massimo Scaglia, the Korean Chim Thack Soh of the Yonsei University of Seoul, and many others. They were all celebrities in infectious and tropical diseases of their time.

They were happy, ingenious, glamorous yet invasive people.

Unfortunately, they have all about disappeared.

Since their work was published mostly in French, I report their precious discoveries to the English world, in the silence of a book.

Although my mother was sometimes exasperated by their fantasies, she liked their company and took an active part in their discussions and projects.

During the summer holidays, I learned to master the technique of tick harvesting, dragging white sheets in the long grass, not too fast, not too slowly. This was the first step of a long process leading to the discovery of a new strain of rickettsia or chlamydia by our scientists. I remember the scene of Mathis, fading more than once, under the dining table in search of one of his favorite lice, which had broken free. The reason why he kept them anchored on his legs, forcing him to wear long socks, was that they had to be fed very carefully and regularly with human blood, to keep their virulence in good shape.

Later I learned that this technique to raise lice was in fact widespread in the scientific world. Antoine van Leewenbeek, a Dutch naturalist, born in 1632, was the first lice breeder ever mentioned in history. With an experimental aim, he decided "to bear for a few days, on an area of his body, what poor people endure on their body during their whole life". He inserted in his sock two beautiful female lice and held these firmly in place with another sock garrotting his knee, for six days. When he removed the garrot to see how the females were, he saw with horror and stupefaction that one female had laid 50 eggs and the other had managed to escape after laying 40 eggs. To learn more about this amazing fecondity, he dissected the remaining female and found in her womb 50 new eggs, nearly matured. He then slipped those eggs into his sock and 10 days later, opening his sock again, he counted 25 little lice, all at different stages of maturation. But at that time he confessed: "disgusted by this vermin, I threw my sock through the window".

Leewenbeek was mainly famous for discovering red cells through lenses of a microscope he designed himself. He observed through those lenses "alive creatures" which later received the name of spermatozoids.

After him, other 'breeders' developed a more sophisticated gadget for their convenience, and to enhance prisoners' detention. One of them was a small box. One side was made of very fine silk and could be attached to the wrist, like a watch, or if preferred, to the calf. In the laboratory of Professor Rudolf Weigl (1883-1957), who was an eminent specialist in exanthematic typhus in Luov, Poland, this kind of breeding was well refined. Fifty staff members were in charge of feeding 400 000 lice, equivalent to 10 000 each.

The problem with lice comes from their metabolism. They only digest blood from humans or monkeys.

Using humans would spare the expense of keeping monkeys.

After his training in Tunis with Nicolle, my father had the opportunity of staying many times at number 6 Sebastian Street, in Cracovia. Until the end of his life, he kept professional links with Poland, where the antigens used for the Micro-agglutination test came from.

In the early Sixties, my father and his colleagues published their work about the relation between rickettsia and multiple sclerosis and other neurological diseases.

One of their mongrels, Zezette, was treated with a lot of consideration because it carried an extraordinary rare strain of rickettsia; a few years ago, its serum was still preciously kept in a Laboratory of the Tropical Institute in Antwerp.

My Sunday morning job was often to take the rectal temperature of a few dozen screaming and smelly guinea pigs. I learned later on that Nicolle was the first one to be able to introduce a thermometer in the guineapigs bums, using a method that I have been taught, which consists of uncurving the lumbar spine and the kidneys of the animal. Without doing so, the thermometer would break inside the poor thing, if you were to introduce it deep enough to be able to read the temperature, and thus cause its death. Because of that, before the use of Nicolle's technique, guineapigs were considered unable to contract typhus.

In my Father's Laboratory, the guineapigs were kept

in two different rooms: the cold room and the warm room. Why did I never question my father about the definite and almost constant difference in body temperature between the two lots of animals? The cold room gave higher readings than the warm room.

The same applied, according to the bric-a-brac of my childhood's memory, to the rooms attributed to the chimpanzees at the laboratory of Bukavu, Kivu. It is only in recent times that I realised that the cold was acting like the stress to weaken their immune defense against the disease they were carrying.

Later on, as I was learning Surgery, I did specialise in chloroforming rats and mice. This is an incredibly delicate task. I had to keep the balance between their inclination to die in the process, and mine to fall asleep after I had nailed them onto a cork theatre plank, sharing their anaesthetic gas. I then had to remove their spleen to compromise their immune resistance for my father's research purposes.

Gradually the rickettsial discussion, the chlamydia and its trachoma, the trypanosomiases, the toxoplasmoses, the debate about the 'cruzine' and its fabulous properties of magic potion, got the better of me. The trypanosom was represented as a kite on a T-shirt received from my father as a post- congress gift. This is probably why their offensive noise irritates me, when they float in the blue sky.

One of my brothers had by then finished his medical studies, and too often for my taste, scientific debates would arise at the family table.

My mother, who grew up in the environment of her father, who also was a famous doctor, and her brothers, who were professors at the university, would take part in these disputes.

I used to run away from this. I found it too heavy and too closed an atmosphere. It was as though nothing else counted in their minds.

Hoping to create a distance between the medical surroundings and me, I presented the entry exam of Les Bois de la Cambre, famous art school in Brussels, to become what I always dreamed of being: an artist. This was a very select school and to enter it was quite an achievment.

However, my Father, exploring my future with, of course, the help of his good friend Paul Giroud, skilfully made me decide otherwise.

Giroud's strong argument in the discussion we had was that I would not be able to buy myself a lot of beautiful little hats because artists are often poor. And I listened to him, with all my feminine intuition, me, who always hated hats. I now only wear the ones I cannot escape, the surgical ones.

After deciding over a period of a few weeks between the different disciplines offered at the university, I entered the Medical School in Louvain, Belgium, as no better choice appeared to be left for me.

I did not know what was waiting for me.

It was difficult to balance life and studies equally.

How could I waste my time loading my brain with all that information? Training the hands to forget life, training the eyes to forget sight, training the lungs to forget breath, dry out the heart, close the ears and force the mind into the belief that it is the only one to exist. I thought it would be easier for me to grow wings like a bird, than to settle into study like a student.

The Physics professor for the first year of Medical School was a man full of charm and vivacity. He was known for his habit, almost maniacal, of choosing one name from a list kept under his arm, and calling it out to verify their presence. The absent would go on a blacklist.

One night in my student bedroom, after having had my usual meal of crisps and duck pâté, I made this professor's head come to life from a lump of clay. I had stolen his face, and, unknown to him, had sculpted his bust. The resemblance was striking. It was two o'clock in the morning, the night of my nineteenth birthday, and I felt like waking up the whole town of Louvain to witness this miracle. I was in a trance, overwhelmed by a feeling of power and completeness.

I am entirely happy like this every time I sculpt a bust, seeing a person appear out of the cold, brown clay. There, in front of me, as if they were coming to life. It was this that sent me into seventh heaven, so much so that I did not care about keeping my sculpture. I could throw it away.

My Physics professor, Mr Capron, thus went the same

way as the others, crumbled to dust, instead of being fired.

There are only two exceptions to this rule: the bust of my father, which I made when I was 15 years old, and which resisted the storms of life for 30 years — when it was shattered, falling from the willing hands of my housekeeper, who was only supposed to dust it; and that of my younger son, Antoine, sculpted when he was almost three years old, and, of course, many thanks to the ceramic oven of a friend.

The seven years that I spent at the University in the superb historical town of Louvain passed too quickly, as do all earthly enchantments. Not only was the architecture splendid, but also the whole town revolved around the students. Les Eaux Douces was a place a little way outside town, situated at the edge of a forest, to where I rode on my bike, until the day it was stolen. Because a bike is an object conceived to be stolen anywhere in the world.

Les Eaux Douces had a riding school, which I attended as often as my meagre financial situation would allow. To ride a horse was a childhood dream and should be just as much a part of education as tennis and bridge.

There was a fine art school, where I would often go in the afternoon, drawing from enduring nude live models, who, for hours posed, tolerantly, without allowing themselves to shiver in the cold of Belgium.

There were also discos at night, which allowed me to

discover the great happiness of getting drunk without wine, of getting intoxicated by dancing to entrancing music.

At that time, I promised myself that I would never stop dancing. From then until the present I have never broken this vow, which kept the uncompromised gravity of my youth. Happily for me, the difference is that I can keep my word without having to go to dances.

When I got home in the early hours to find my bed, I would regularly cross the look out at an angle to the ideal students smelling of fresh soap, who were going to lectures, their hair neat and tidy and briefcases under the arms. Briefcases packed with all the right books that I had not yet bought, and in all likelihood, would never buy.

In fact, it is amazing how much memory you can save if you are forced by lack of time. And what is even more amazing is that you get practically the same result. It is clear that the hare runs faster than the tortoise, because of its physical constitution, even if Monsieur De La Fontaine tried to prove it wrong.

During the time of swotting before finals exams, my whole family suffered, including the noisy grey parrot that I locked in a spare room of the house rather than strangle it, because he could not understand he had to shut his big mouth.

I retreated into my father's office.

I gave my mother grey hair because I asked her to

explain my English chemistry book.

My mother was a remarkable woman, beautiful, clever, at ease with language or any other subject. It is from her that I inherited my passion for art, luxurious tastes, and love of cooking. Her phenomenal brain guided me from capital letters to small letters, from Latin to Algebra, from Greek to Science, passing through English on the way. Assuredly, the Diploma of Medicine should have been awarded to her.

Without my mother, I would never have become a doctor. Without her help and that of charitable friends, who took pity on the dreamer that I was, and gave me books. Without all this, my studies would have followed the course of the Titanic.

I do not think that my husband would have married me had he met me during that period in my life. He was a good, systematic, organised student. One day, when we first met, he showed me his textbooks, neatly arranged on the shelves, full of intelligent notes and comments. I had never realised that someone could have so many books. The medical competence he acquired during his studies was far superior to mine, and I was lucky to have his encyclopaedic brain at my disposal.

After completing the seven years of Medicine, I started to specialise in Surgery, but not because it was an irresistible vocation.

As usual in my life, my best guide for decisions was my instinct.

I was rather attracted by the incredible skill and the

vaporous eyes — with a hunter's look — of the surgeon I chose as mentor in this field, Mr Edouard Aubry.

But I also definitely trusted that by enrolling in a different discipline all together, the wall I had built between rickettsial diseases and myself was comfortable, anyway, at this stage of my life.

I regarded those studies for my own education only; I had in mind that I would never work professionally, as my mother did not, and that I would soon return to my art and parties.

I will never regret my choice. I needed this period of strict discipline and intensive work for my later work ethic, to get out of my laziness and nocturnal habits.

At times, night and day we had to stitch. The warm blood was drying on skin and gown. The cries and sorrow of the wounded resonated in my head. Progressively, the virtue of concentration, focus and endurance instead of failing, increased under this regime. It is only by stitching that one learns how to stitch. I really loved those hours, passed in silence that could be cut by a knife, close to the genius of surgical technique. Or was he an artist with a lancet instead of a brush in his hand?

It was like muted music for a ballet, performed by rubber-gloved fingers, which crossed, touched, enlaced, rested and took flight again.

These precise movements, fast and co-ordinated, would hold observers breathless, as if it was a premier performance. One forgot the acrid smell of blood, the tension, the tiredness, the hunger and thirst.

Nothing existed other than the work in progress in this human factory. The satisfaction received was as intense as the work was hard.

To know this rapture with surgery is an incredible privilege for which I will always thank my dear mentor. This genius, by allowing me the access, gave me the gift for hard work and concentration that I never would have found in any other school. I transferred his likeness, too, in a clay bust during one of those nights when I was in touch with heaven. I saw his grave serious expression each time I removed the damp cloth, intended to slow down the drying process, from his face. I would be intimidated by every glance at his clay face. It looked so much like him.

One day, my husband and I moved to a cottage in the mountains close to the Ardennes Forest, on my mentor's advice. A steep stair gave access to the house. The bust never came inside for reasons I never asked myself. It slowly melted under the constant drizzle that gives Belgium its green salad look in its faded sepia.

CHAPTER 4:

MY SOUTH AFRICAN SURROUNDINGS

"Africa has been for us and for ever
A fascinating and imperishable source of
investigation."
—*Prof Dr Rud Geigy*—
Horizons 80.

In 1981, I came to South Africa to complete my surgical degree. The plan was to stay there for one year and then go back to the open Belgian market. Of course, my husband accompanied me. He is a medical doctor specialised in pathology and was appointed to work for the South African Institute for Medical Research.

Pregnant with our eldest son just before our arrival in South Africa, in the middle of January 1981 — Jean-Baptiste celebrates his 21th birthday on 3 July 2002 — I was refused my job as an assistant in paediatric surgery, for which I had been previously accepted. I was devastated by this extreme measure.

Who was this man capable of dismissing me without even testing my capabilities?

This swine did not want any of my pearls.

Did he not know that a pregnancy is not carried in the hands?

What traces of curbing of labour or of surgical indecency did he detect in round bellies?

Oh, how arrogant he was! What an obsolete mentality!

Added to this, this medieval rudeness did not seem to disturb my colleagues more than the presence of a beggar on the street corner. What a country of machos.

From operating theatres to corridors, as transfusions proceeded drop by drop, from surgeons to nurses, from streams to floods, from breakers to surf, the rumour grumbled in xenophobic notes that the Belgian brood-mare should return to her stable.

"Of course, this is not the first time that this has been done to us. In the first place, there is their accent that is completely incomprehensible. Scissors!" cried the surgeon to his assistant, who was compelled to hear him.

"If there had been only that. Do you remember the

one whose diploma was not even acceptable? Be careful, Miss. Do not dab dry tissue; you will cause it to bleed. You are not following the operation." His tone was as sharp as his bistoury.

Apart from the story about the apparently illegal diploma, I perceived a few shivers around this table.

"Yes, I remember that well. It happened a year ago. He came from India, I think. Apparently he had bought his diploma. And this other man, the one from Luxembourg, who arrived three months after the anticipated date," a laconic voice continued. "Now then, the skin please," the impatient hand of this same voice stressed.

"They come here to acquire experience. Where they come from, they are only allowed to watch. We will not hold it against you if you are fast," resumed somebody in an oppressive tone.

"I have not been caught in a long time. It is you again, the table assistant. Why are you making the same mistakes as yesterday? This is really incredible. Aspiration is for here and now and not for tomorrow." Involuntary trembling followed this declaration.

"Me neither. I notified them by letter that they should not make any more propositions. They might as well stay at home. As if one needed their services. I did not ask you for a Mc Gills." The violent embezzlement of the ill-chosen forceps tore the operating space and the assistant in multiple confusions.

In these cases, it is never the patients that are torn.

77

Only, everything does not always occur between silk and velvet.

Some virtuosos of surgery do not manage to maintain themselves in the ring. They then get undressed, allow water to run, change their gloves and the curtain is raised.

"As if we did not have enough problems with our own locals. No, do not cut the thread so short. One would think that you are set on segmenting the knots." Cold sweats were guaranteed at this table, as well as a growing hatred for this pretentious mocker.

"Oh, these foreigners. We will never be rid of them. Come on, do not fall asleep on the retractors. A bit of effort please." There, muscular cramps invade the forearms.

"A few of them are brilliant, despite everything."

As usual, admiration is given to the integrals.

"Agreed, but these remain the exception…"

It seemed senseless for me to continue in this risky place, where racism seemed to be a conventional and polymorph pastime.

Why did I leave Belgium with its substantial offers?

A striking raid is not the shortest distance between two points.

Was my entire universe about to give way due to some professional fuss?

With Eeyore's (the donkey in Winnie the Pooh) state of mind, but with rational reasons for being so, I lounged the streets of Hillbrow, speculating that I could always throw myself into polemic study. Alexandra Road, its bustling charms lost, opened onto the Metropolitan, in which the apartment that we were renting was found — which was on the 14th floor. It was in this building that most of the French and Belgian doctors began their careers in South Africa.

We would most probably have been on the 13th floor if it had existed, I thought, allowing myself to sink into a corrosive melancholy.

Stretched out on the edge of the pool of our skyscraper, I waited for my husband so we could share our troubles over lunch. I did not wait long: he lost his job at about 10:30 am, half an hour after I had lost mine, as his English was not up to scratch.

"Have English lessons," They had advised him as they handed him a contact number. He showed this to me to prove that this was not a fantasy. I told him about my own disappointments. They seemed to be worse now that I had heard my husband's news: no contact number existed to solve a pregnancy.

A couple was seated by the pool, their feet in search of coolness in this late morning of a South African mid-January, so weighed down by sad stories and moist heat that they had appetite and legs suspended.

They were in the shape of temporary disincarnation. Time scattered itself in disorganised minutes as a defeated army is folded up after defeat. The air was scorching, painful for the lungs, and the sunset was not going to rectify the situation.

That was the beginning.

Our escapade to the tropics had failed.

Did we now have to rid ourselves of the old Citroen that was not roadworthy anyway, and dispel ourselves forever in the swamps of Belgium?

My father, as always, was the charismatic solution.

How could I have, even for an instant, forgotten this fundamental taboo?

His scientific connections had more influence than any added Rotary or Lion's Club. After a phone call to my magical begetter, Professor Gear invited us for dinner instead of being unwelcome individuals. My father and this man were old friends. What is more, James Gear had been the director of the South African Institute for Medical Research.

This was a stroke of fortune of the first order.

Pyramids are found everywhere.

We obviously needed more than just a pipette to dilute this degradation.

But for mysterious reasons costly to the human being, the straw often appears to be larger than the pole. Stormy weather dominates over the rays of sunshine and we almost missed our second chance.

"Please take your seats," he said as he opened the door of his Ford, "I am inviting you to dinner." Their superb house in the suburb of Houghton offered a serene atmosphere, fitting the situation, which perfectly matched the succulent meal prepared by Mrs Gear. She was a charming hostess who had prepared a dish especially for the daughter of her dear Jean. Well fed and relieved, we signed the guest book and took leave, thanking our new guardian angels.

Access to the Medical Institute reopened warmly, regarding my husband Patrick's aptitude, now considered under a different light. He was soon on his way to exciting haematological adventures, with the aid of an English dictionary.

As for me, my itinerary took another course and I found out that most seemingly positive long-term trajectories balanced out negative ones. I was not long in mourning for employment.

We had to make provision for English lessons, of course. Anne was the name of our teacher. She was pretty and blonde, tall and jovial, pronouncing the word 'cute' with scrunched up lips like a hen on the verge of laying an egg, and asking us to do the same.

Three weeks later my husband, thanks to his competency and undeniable talent for languages, though hidden, presented his first work before a group of doctors struck dumb by his progress.

Amongst the audience sat Penny, the chief medical technologist.

"Who is that young man? How charming, how good looking." Nothing more was needed to start a life-long friendship.

The bliss of living beneath the rays of the sun quickly engulfed my mind and body.

"This country has the greatest climate in the world,

with the longest hours of sunshine and the most pleasant temperatures," my mother affirmed. She had visited South Africa on several occasions since 1940.

"As soon as the temperature exceeds the desired range, a rain shower overthrows the situation. And the delicious aromas that follow disperse any flies that may be," she guaranteed optimistically, yet wisely, omitting to name the forces regularly unfurled to do so. She possessed a perfectly finished talent for cooling the heat into freshness, and for transforming clamminess into rich perfume. Here was her description of the season incorrectly called 'rainy season', as it would stand for a diminutive of the 'thunderstorms season'.

The horizon before had renewed values. Values, which were not unknown to me. The adjustment happened without any misfortune. Light transformed all that it touched into sublime paintings.

The beauty was as obvious as the last argument of a polemic would be to a controversial person. Even the simplest of sparrows made me catch my breath with admiration. Its well assembled, glistening body, a rhyme held in its beak, seemed to share nothing with its cousins from the north — but a common name. I have reread this sentence after having observed these little creatures once again, and have concluded that my first thoughts were correct.

There were superb trees with trunks peeled by winds heavy with succulent scents. Their name, the blue gum for Eucalyptus, reminded me of candy.

I watched with fascination the explosions of the unruly cascades of bougainvilleas. Those were of a purple as discrete as a volcano in effervescence.

The giant moonflowers were seductive, draped in white like dumb Callas awakened by some secret and silent message.

The African women defy Newton as they file out in luminous colours on a footpath in the Berg, rigged up with a bundle of firewood on their heads, a cherub knotted up on their backs and a gigantic pair of breasts swaying heavily with the rhythm of the bow.

The African children were captivating, their heads seemingly adorned with miniature hills where sugar-cane was planted, after a tractor had hoed them.

The girls were graceful with their sun-washed doe eyes, their eyelids beating in a Walt Disney fashion.

The vegetation was abundant and majestic, containing seriously venomous snakes and scorpions without star signs, identical to poisonous gifts of the heavens.

All this rendered more bearable the consumer-orientated society, which nearly drowned me in Belgium.

Here, there were so many shocking events that I began to forget my enforced membership of this totalitarian society that was so focused on perishable delights.

From where did all these scenic creations come?

Surely the word 'tropics' implied 'luxury'.

The warmth was as gentle as a therapeutic recital.

The rain unearthed fragrances that it alone was capable of defining.

The extraordinary invasive gambol of colours imprinted itself into my receptive brain. Opportunistic imprints that left perpetual scars.

As I did not develop any immunity against these sublime and boisterous surroundings, I began to paint. I penetrated a momentous universe already existing under the title of passion, rage, intoxication and bliss.

The walls began to be covered with paintings. Some were offered to family members, with or without their consent. Others were for the friends whom I valued, worthy of my assortment without worrying about their contingency. The gynaecologist whom I had to consult those days and the family dentist seemed only delighted to spend time and trouble for nothing but a few landscapes. Dogs used to nibble corners, tomcats marked their territories and the parrot sometimes sharpened his beak on non-unattended pictures.

I found an alternative to surgery.

I refused to be transformed into a salt statue, by looking back one last time on the closed doors of the operating theatre. I worshipped another god.

Beneath my hair that became sun-bleached, and with my skin once again tanned by the eternal idol, I regained that African princess of the happy days.

Of course, there were thunderstorms now and then.

Of course, we had not come for the political climate, or for the growing violence, or for any other scandal.

Of course, we did not drink tea if given the choice and the men's eyes were as functional as their words.

It was true that life under the African sun was an antagonist, regarding the medical careers that we had envisioned for ourselves.

Yet the thought of returning permanently to the European sheep-pen sent shivers down my spine. Was I that much in love with chameleons?

How does one find a balance point between boring security and blissful peril?

On a lighter note, our choice became nothing more than an unravelled fan: planted in African humus, our roots had established an affinity that was as autonomous as it was irrevocable.

Thus we decided to throw ourselves into the next station forecasted for Franco-Belgian doctors: house-sitting. This involved occupying a residence whose owners were travelling overseas. We landed up with a house whose Afrikaner architecture was striking.

In the calm street of the suburb bordered with plantains, stood an automobile per house, preferably a white obsolete model, yet immaculate despite the dust, good performance in this hot and dry climate. Its presence betrayed the neighbourhood's identity.

A dozen labourers, black, since this specification is necessary regarding this scene taken from this damned country in the 80s, were stretching their glistening muscles over pickaxes beneath the liquid sun. This scene could have been one of Sekoto's masterpieces, except that they never lifted their arms simultaneously, which is indispensable for a Herculean image of a mass in action, so well rendered by this artist.

The dwelling's entrance, the 'stoep', was as solid as dog kennel. There was the hint of a Boer's silhouette, with his rectangular beard and a mug of steaming coffee sheltered from the sun's offence. Once beyond the sill, the pine floorboards gave away the comings and goings of the hypothetically large wife, who was also the author of the cup of coffee and who hastily, added the overlooked newspaper. The rooms, small and dim, contrasted oddly with their plastered ceilings, which might have been sculpted for an opera.

The whole of it was encircled by a small garden that had a view onto Galatea Street.

The toilet was situated at the bottom of the garden, a detail that can be neglected if one does not consider the rigour of winter at 1 680m above sea level, and that I was in the late stages of pregnancy. Pregnant or not, all the women of my street shared the same fate, night and day, of using the luxurious gutters.

On termination of the lease, taken by one completely smitten by this country, and as out of fashion as a cow intent on remaining multicoloured, we bought our own house.

With architecture as unsure as the previous house's, it was pitched in a similar neighbourhood. The compulsory stoep was at the back of the house this time, overlooking a clear blue pool, which, with facilities within reach of the bedrooms, fully justified the purchase of this house.

My son was then three months old. He was an adorable baby, vigorous, blond with dark eyes, bubbling with laughs and tears. As he was growing without any problems, disregarding his untreatable insomnia at bedtime, which he is still making up for today, I decided to start working again.

Coronation Hospital was discovered a few kilometres away. I was accepted at once. Only some months later, the superintendent had the sense to ignore, from a professional point of view, that I was about to give birth to my daughter Aurélie.

I thus worked there three years during which I learned to appreciate the Malaysians, Indians and Mulattos — all assembled beneath the same roof by the now dying Apartheid regime.

During the immoderate work periods in a violent and chaotic climate, I made friends in the medical profession of whom I do not know the colour and who are closer to me than my own brothers.

Unbelievable Apartheid.

Inhuman solution legalised to solve a human problem. Fear generates hate.

Even for someone like me who was not feeling concerned by this situation, it did not pass unnoticed. It reinforced my natural aversion to politics and its actors.

My skin's colour automatically ranked me in the

guilty camp.

To reject the whole country because of its current government seemed to me like a snobbish child's play, rather than a brilliant action. It was not in any case my manner to take sides.

My powerlessness turned silent, 'deaf' and 'blind'. I used to ignore conventions. I did not want to realise that my son was the only white at school, and I became a member of the tearoom I was not supposed to enter.

And yet, I could not ignore that there were not many 'blacks' behind the wheel. Patients visited the hospital by foot and for all sorts of pathological problems.

However many of them appeared after a blood bath with axe, dagger or knife wounds. These were disinfected, explored and sutured. The cold steel was laid out in a basket, waiting for its owner. One day, as I was busy writing in a file, I felt the cold of a gun between my shoulders, because I omitted to give the ammunition back. Life was not interrupted for so little.

With the exception of the one who, after having walked to the hospital, had the axe removed that was planted in his skull. Driven in well above the periostium during a fit of passion, without a shadow of indulgence, the function of the axe was modified to become a vital haemostatic. My colleague had just enough time to marvel at the still-standing patient's resilience, before laying him down for eternity and setting him free from his foreign body.

Nowadays, young doctors have to confront the

damage caused by the Kalyshnikovs, more accurately AK 47s. Every century has its gold.

After the birth of my daughter, I decided to open a medical practice, where I hoped to have chief control over a life that, according to me, should have a less spectacular demeanour.

A few months passed before I had to take on my first cadaver, stranded in the doorway seeking aid after a night that was just too hurtful. This was the first curtain drawn of many, for the same theme song. Was this the reason for the interruption of my five-month pregnancy?

My life seems to be continually in suspension.

But happiness is difficult to disarm.

One year later, Antoine, our third child, appeared.

My husband, until then occupied by his post in internal medicine at Coronation Hospital, took over the general practice. Still working with him a few sessions a week, I went back to surgery and discovered the hermetical world of the Afrikaaners in the theatre of a private clinic.

In those days, occasionally, in my South African practice, I met patients with the diagnosis of myalgic encephalomyelitis (ME).

My father had never heard of it, nor had my colleagues in Belgium and France.

It must have been a British creation.

Although many practitioners refused to recognise this badly-defined newly-emerging condition, others accused viruses such as coxsackie, cytomegalovirus and Epstein Barr virus as being the cause of it. Stress or depression was also blamed.

Eventually these patients were treated with antidepressants, sedatives, cocktails of vitamins, electrolytes and minerals, anti-inflammatories, or gamma globulins extracted from human tissue. If this did not work, the patient was given electro convulsive therapy.

At this time, ME, more often called chronic fatigue syndrome (CFS), is not yet a clear entity. This condition is stuck with its own definition, relying on symptomatic criteria established by certain physicians in charge, or considered to be psychosomatic by others.

No wonder that, because of this confused start in the medical world, CFS has and will still need a lot of pruning to be rehabilitated and considered as a real disease.

The incoherence of the approach to CFS was obvious to my Cartesian mind, but I did not care much, as it was not exactly my field of practice.

I was not really perturbed by the despondency of those patients until I met Pauline.

Pauline was a professional horse-rider and had a well-established, very busy riding school. She had a husband and three children .The whole family soon became our patients as they were living close to our surgery.

My husband Patrick has never been able to live without being surrounded by horses; his cowboy style is one of his charms that made me fall in love with him. He had to get rid of his horse in Belgium, to follow me to South Africa.

So, as soon as we could, this injustice was repaired by the purchase of an Arab mare, being the horse of his dreams in those days. Her name was Silvido Dorena. She was beautiful but badly assembled and, as it happens in packages of travelling agencies, she was pregnant.

Obviously the start of a long story, something like the one of the never-ending Russian dolls.

We started to look for accommodation, as close as possible to the surgery, so that the happy owner would be able to visit her as often as possible, during his little spare time.

Then innocently, Pauline came into my life, offering to stable a horse, but actually throwing me into a new rickettsial storm.

She was the missing link between my past and my future.

She was a serious dressage rider and her husband was doing well in business.

As she said: "Life was really good. The road to success was afore me, naught could befall me."

But, suddenly, what is it about a Monday, when she wanted to get herself going to start the day? She could not. She felt awfully weak. It was flu, she thought and crawled back to bed. In a few days time, she would be better. But she was worse. One week later, she was admitted to the hospital under the supervision of a physician for diagnostic tests.

She wrote: "They prodded, poked, drew blood, tested down the top end, tested up the bottom end ... nothing."

Absolutely nothing. No diagnosis and not better.

Four days later, she was home again, bedridden, despondent and confused. My suggestion was that she was suffering from a rickettsial infection. This was logical to me, because of her symptomatology of tiredness and body aches, and because of her occupation.

Therefore the Weil Felix test was performed on Pauline's serum. This was the routine test for rickettsial diagnostic purposes in those days and in this country. One week later, the results came back negative. One week later, six months later, one year later, four years later, the test was repeated and stayed negative.

In that period of time, I did not know much about the different diagnostic tests available for rickettsioses. I had no inclination to read textbooks. So the opinions of the Lenette book of microbiology about the Weil Felix test was unknown to me: "...do not use the Weil Felix test, the result will mean nothing at the best and may cause confusion at the worst. By far the most useful and practical rickettsial agglutination test that has been developed is the Micro-agglutination test. The simplicity of the Micro-agglutination test and the generally good reproducibility of results are strong recommendations for its general use, when appropriate antigens become commercially available. No antigens for the Micro-agglutination test are available from the Centre for Disease Control or from any commercial source at this time."

I also had not heard about J E Mc Dade's opinion: "The Centre for Disease Control has established criteria for positivity for the various serological tests. Fourfold rises in titre detected by any technique (Weil Felix excepted) are considered evidence of rickettsial infections."

In a similar way, no chance of my having read the following: "The Weil–Felix test, uses various strains of Proteus. Because it lacks both sensitivity and specificity, it should no longer be used."

It would also have been a help to know that: "Advances in a few top laboratories are only poorly reflected in developing countries i.e. in regions with the highest occurrence of rickettsial diseases. The lack of specific antigens as well as of skilled workers makes it possible to survive the use of Weil–Felix (WF) reaction."

Let's just add a letter to the editor of the American Journal of Medicine, written in 1986, under the title: The Weil–Felix test is archaic and misleading.

Indeed, I had not realised that using that way of testing, Pauline stood no chance of getting a decent answer to her query of rickettsial infection.

Pauline then tested positive for glandular fever and for coxsackie viruses. She was diagnosed as suffering from depression, due to her stressful life-style. Gamma globulin injections were used, then antidepressants and beta-blockers to calm her anxiety and her palpitations.

Despite all that, she was virtually confined to her room between teaching sessions, sitting in a chair beside the arena so that she did not exert too much energy. People were wondering about her.

During this period she did not consult me, as she was under the supervision of a top muscle specialist who was also known as the leading ME specialist in South Africa. He performed a muscle biopsy. The diagnosis given to her was the presence of 'tombstones', meaning dead areas in the muscles. Potassium and magnesium were given for pins and needles in her hands.

Her symptoms ranged from a terrible exhaustion exacerbated by exercise, severe muscle weakness and pain, heart palpitations, bouts of depression, headaches and repeated urinary infections.

Her specialist suggested she should join the quickly-growing group of ME sufferers, soon labelled with an even more disgraceful name, Yuppie flu.

But was that a diagnosis? Was there a treatment? Where was the prognosis? What was the cause?

Despite repeating the Weil Felix test several times during the four years that her disease lasted, keeping in mind my suggestion of a possible rickettsial infection, the results stayed inconclusive.

To keep her business going, she bought herself a four-wheel motorcycle. Her husband learned to do the shopping, and her children learned how to pass by their mother quickly, as to avoid her endless orders.

Months became years, and Pauline, more or less non-ambulatory, was learning to adapt to this situation with a disciplined lifestyle to insure enough energy for the major expenses of her daily life.

Her appendix was removed and this put an end to her chronic urinary infection, probably due to the fact that the infected appendix was truly flirting with her bladder.

She took part in a television programme about ME patients, where she illustrated how sufferers could cope with the disability.

One day, out of desperation, Pauline asked me about the possibility of sending her serum to my father for testing for rickettsial infection.

Two phone calls later, one to my father and one to the post office, the serum was on its way to Belgium.

I had no idea how one unique serum sample could change the rest of my life, pushing me out of my comfortable routine.

The result of the test done by my father showed strong antibodies against Rickettsia prowazeki and Rickettsia mooseri and no antibodies against Rickettsia conori and Coxiella burnetti or against Neo-rickettsia chlamydia Q18 group responsible for recurrent abortions in sheep.

In sheep only?

My father commented about the frequency of these

mixed infections.

We discussed Pauline's symptoms. My father considered the positivity against two different strains of rickettsia, together with the symptoms as being a chronic rickettsial infection and he suggested a protocol of treatment.

In an atmosphere of mutual scepticism, Pauline started her tetracycline treatment just a week before Christmas.

Seventy-two hours later, she phoned to tell me she was qualitatively better.

Her mind filled with doubt, she risked going to the nearby shopping centre, more to test her own ability than to face the rest of the world and the Christmas songs.

Her family, who escorted her, could not believe this sight and Pauline could not believe her legs. I thought maybe she exaggerated the improvement of her disease, or maybe she previously overrated the severity of her symptoms.

Was it not too early to consider such progress?

Later on, I read in a pharmacology textbook (Goodman et al) that after a single oral dose of tetracycline, peak plasma concentrations are attained in two to four hours.

Two weeks later, Pauline recovered her efficiency on her best show jumper.

Being of a sociable and energetic nature, this spectacular healing did not pass unnoticed.

The local equestrian press interviewed Pauline and consequently her good doctor had to apply for an official export permit, which she received promptly, to send more serum to Belgium. Indeed, numerous patients wanted to be tested for rickettsial and chlamydial infections by the Micro-agglutination test, because of Pauline's impressive recovery.

Having been exposed for as long as I can remember to my father's scientific approach and work, I never doubted the value of my diagnosis but still I could not but be astonished by the results of my treatment: why were my patients constantly improving?

Thereafter, by word of mouth, the number of patients treated by me and doing well on this treatment grew very quickly. They generally presented with similar complaints, such as fatigue, pain in their muscles and joints, and depression. The results of my father kept on showing a well-built positivity for rickettsial antibodies in 90% of the cases.

It was now becoming obvious that I was facing a new entity: it was that impressive mass of rejected patients thrown into the loneliness of a no-man's land named Yuppie flu, ME or post viral fatigue syndrome by the medical fraternity.

I felt the symptoms of these patients were due to rickettsial infection. But was it so simple?

Here, as elsewhere, very little was said about rickettsial illnesses. Tick bite fever was the only disease considered to result from a tick bite. This condition was treated with a low dosage of tetracycline for five days and the patient was supposed to recover forever. Mention was sometimes made of Q fever, thought to be a serious condition, but rarely developed. In the student books of medical schools, two pages covered the subject. Obviously not enough to become familiar with the wide pathology it could produce.

This is probably why nobody before me ever thought of the link between that CFS condition and the rickettsial diseases.

I had never considered the danger of speaking about it and now I had no choice. It was too late to go backwards. The loop was now closing on a world that I had avoided all my life, and which was coming back inexorably. I had to go forward.

My father sent me the medical literature I had banished from my bookshelf for years. I was caught in a trap. I could not resist writing my first medical paper to share with others my discovery. The title I chose was: ME, a new name for an old disease.

Proudly I sent the manuscript to the South African Medical Journal. The reply did not take long: "No room for your article in our journal". I could not obtain any explanation from the editor, who was repeatedly unavailable for comment.

It was not enough to dishearten my obstinate nature.

In association with Dr Philippe Bottero, a disciple of Dr Paul Legag and my father, we convened in the old family home in Anvers, Belgium, where the ambiance was filled by my parents' presence to discuss a paper to be published in the premier English medical journal, The Lancet.

As a family friend and professor of Medical Protozoology at the London School of Hygiene and Tropical Medicine at the University of London, Prof P C Garnham was acquainted with this publication to be, and congratulated me. Nevertheless, he expressed doubt about this new revolutionary idea.

The answer from The Lancet confirmed his opinion: a double blind study was necessary before publishing this article, to prevent any equivocal conclusion.

Using this method, I was supposed to match patients of the same age, the same sex, diagnose them, get the same result and then treat half of them with my antibiotic, and the other half with a placebo regime, consisting of tablets having the same appearance, but containing pure powder. The patients selected for this study were supposed to sign an agreement that they were willing to take part in an experimental study, and would not be informed of the nature of their treatment. Then, I should have to compare the progress of the two different groups and report it.

That was the only way, according to the letter I received, to get credit for the accuracy of my treatment and to have access to a publication in The Lancet.

Not only was this impossible to apply in a private surgery, but the respect that I have for my patients will always prevent me from practicing this experimental method. As my treatment came after positive verification of rickettsial infection, I was not just treating fatigue with antibiotics, but I was following the numerous guidelines for combating the presence of intracellular organisms. Therefore, from the start I was practising a kind of 'evidence based medicine', as opposed to 'experimental medicine'.

This was my second cold shower.

Coincidently, a few years later, in a 'letter to the editor', The Lancet suggested "post Q fever syndrome as a new name for CFS" (April 1996 edition). Indeed, Q fever is caused by Coxiella burnetti, a type of rickettsia. The Q stands for query, as a simple question mark for the cause of this fever.

For the time being I then forgot about scientists with their slow and prudent steps and concentrated on my patients, who were progressing well and spreading world of their cure.

They were farmers, ecologists, riders, hikers, golf players, pet lovers, outdoor fanatics, and young men coming back from the army service. They came from everywhere.

I was then asked to open clinics in Port Elizabeth, in Cape Town, then in Pietermaritzburg. I soon also had patients from Europe, Australia and the United States.

All of them presented with the same symptoms where fatigue was predominant; they had antibodies to the intracellular infective bacteria, rickettsia, chlamydia and mycoplasma, and reacted similarly to the same antibiotic therapy.

Not only were they feeling better but also their blood results were improving or normalising, and eventually the patients were going back to their earlier performances, forgetting about their previous medical and drug shopping.

In 1992, Pauline again was the subject of a further television programme in the series called 50/50 and gave a follow-up on the first interview.

This time she explained her new condition with her theme song: "Call it ME, call it scrambled eggs disease, nevertheless I am cured .The proof of the pudding is in the eating".

Now, whether I wished it or not, I became of interest to the TV producers.

An amiable producer informed me that although the majority of my patients were better and testified to it, there was growing opposition from some of my South African medical colleagues.

The television programme showed a group of virologists, dressed in white behind their microscopes, talking about me with clear reservations. Pauline, fully convinced of her recovery, was pictured in great condition, riding her horse in her arena.

The crew took some shots of me, riding Salut, my grey horse, or displaying some of my paintings, which were supposedly reflecting the perplexity of my behaviour: what credibility is left to a female doctor, who not only rides a horse, but is also an artist?

After the TV producer's visit to the Virology Institute, the ambiance of the production had changed from friendly to hostile.

The film produced was one sided, and not on my side. It failed to emphasise the scientific basis to my diagnosis, it failed to acknowledge the known incidence of rickettsial diseases in South Africa, and most of all it failed to present all the facts. It is remarkable how often in our society and through history experts say initially "there is no basis to that belief", then "it is not to be trusted", followed by "it is obvious that...".

50/50 was aired on 7 June 1992. It sounded strangely like a declaration of war.

In April 1993, the South African Medical and Dental Council sent me a letter by registered mail, which my distraught husband handed to me. It started: "You are guilty of improper and disgraceful conduct ..."

CHAPTER 5:

I STAND ACCUSED: A MEDICAL INQUIRY THAT RESEMBLED A COURT CASE

"Nobody is your enemy.
Everyone is your instructor."
—*Arab proverb*—

"You are guilty of improper and disgraceful conduct," the Medical Council impeached me and charged me on April 20, 1993. Without any investigation.

The charge sheet said that I had treated specific people, whose names I had never heard, in places I had never been to, in such a manner, as I had never thought of.

The adjectives used in this letter included: "unjustifiable, unscientific, unwarranted, risky, harmful, unreliable, outdated, primitive, meaningless, misleading, medically irrelevant, exploitation, advertising, damaging the standard and the reputation of the profession to which you belong, during 1991, 1992 and 1993".

So, I must have hurt someone, or even killed someone?

Why did that patient not come back to me with the problem? Surely, I could have helped, and if not, at least I would have known. How could something major have happened to one of my patients without my being informed?

The charge mentioned the names of 10 patients having been harmed by my treatment. On closer examination, only half of these had come to see me. Others were not my patients. The injuries they had suffered from, according to them, had been nausea, occasional vomiting and headaches, while they were being treated.

I was reassured, but then, was that all I was guilty of? How could an unsettled stomach possibly start a legal procedure?

It was not necessary to read the 40 pages attached to the accusation pages to realise how perception can fool you. I had thought I was doing a really good job, as my patients were recovering so well. In the meantime, some well-known people practising the same profession as mine were expressing their opinions using these words: My treatment was dangerous. My diagnosis was wrong. My fees were exorbitant. My father's test was 'bogus'. I was practising an itinerant type of medicine.

By contravening the provisions of Rule 1 and Rule 7 of the Ethical Rules, I was acting illegally and unscrupulously.

In this charge, it was said that I was consulting and treating large groups of patients in Johannesburg, Port Elizabeth, Cape Town, Howick and East London.

Reading it was enough to give a solid vertigo to any mother of three young children, never mind the lazy person I am by nature. I still have never been to Howick or East London.

In short, the picture I presented was that of a lost woman in a country steeped in religious conservatism.

The point was made about my being a Belgium national and therefore a foreigner and, of course, my qualifications were not South African. It was also stipulated that my diagnostic tests did not emanate from their pathological centres, but from an unknown laboratory in Belgium. For that reason, recommendations were given to consider the results with the necessary awareness.

An attached document explained that: "the treatment of Dr Jadin is not scientific, and designed to attract and exploit the mass of those sufferers despondent enough to seek any kind of help".

The evidence was to be presented in this way. It would retain this form until proven to the contrary. For this reason, it would take over three years of investigations: first, the preliminary meetings with lawyers, when I became familiar with the skyscrapers of Pretoria; then, long sessions before the Medical Council situated at the end of Vermeulen Street in Arcadia, the administrative area of Pretoria.

The Medical Council operated mainly in two sections.

The administrative section, a kind of effervescent beehive where switchboard operators seemed to be tied to high-voltage charged receivers, and where numerous machines were continuously unrolling metres of faxes.

The other section consisted of the two 'in camera' rooms, which were very similar to each other but for size.

With a heart as leaden as my legs, I proceeded to this select and mysterious den. The seat of honour, where my future was going to be decided, was reserved for me. Subdued lighting, luxurious materials, long faces, spastic microphones, purring typewriters. Constant whisperings, words designed to trap, cold air-conditioning, and a feeling of hostility towards the guilty one. Added to this, always the smell of wax polish permeating the room. This could be the reason why aspirin was commonly in use.

The official session eventually began on the 9th of February 1995.

The sitting committee was composed of three

members. Fortunately, on this occasion, I could link faces and names and immediately recognised the Chairman Dr S, who was a close collaborator and friend of the main plaintiff, Dr A S. Indeed, I remember him, sitting with Prof Gear at a meeting at the Institute of X where I had been invited to discuss my treatment, sometime in 1993. I realised that with him at the head of the committee, I would not stand much chance. My lawyers agreed with me, and they asked that he be taken off the case.

The session was then adjourned and postponed to another date, in order to have time to find a new chairman. Professor FJM was appointed and the hearing commenced. I attended a session three to four days a week, three to four times a year, up until January 1997.

Initially, charges fell like raindrops on my head while I stood silently by, noting my comments and passing them on to my lawyers, who instantly read them. It was very difficult. Later, I was allowed to answer the prosecutor's questions directly. Often these questions fell weightily, provoking me to answer with humour. The tension began to dissolve in laughter.

The media was always present, supporting the opposition, and reports appeared in newspapers. The names of my accusers were published.

Who were the authors of those charges?

According to the newspapers, they were general

practitioners, specialists in biology, surgery, pharmacy and other disciplines. They had gathered against me under the auspices of a most irate virologist.

The first article in the Sunday Times, published in August 1992, was so startling that even the contemporary rugby scandal lost a bit of its allure. It reported that:

"Many doctors claim the treatment she gives is inappropriate and possibly harmful", and a little further on: "Local doctors say the test done by Dr Jadin has been overtaken by more accurate and sophisticated tests and is no longer used in South Africa". Dr BS claimed that "the benefits of tetracyclines were speculative and anecdotal and the associated risks were mild to life threatening".

Further, Prof JT, Prof HK, Dr FS and Dr AS all added their comments to the report published in the Sunday Times, referring to me as a "self-styled yuppie flu expert facing charges of disgraceful conduct after allegedly exploiting patients medically and financially and prescribing unsafe doses of antibiotics", and also to "the obsolete test of her father".

Some months later, a journalist reported that: "E O'D, a Cape Town advertising agency media planner, alleged that she was told to have her blood drawn by a laboratory and to post it to Belgium, labelling the contents as cosmetics to overcome regulations for sending blood out of the country." When I managed to put a face to the name, I well remembered a neurotic woman living in Cape Town. At every consultation, she and her friend embarked on lengthy arguments that always encroached on my time schedule. Complaints made by both these women to the Medical Council, that they had become increasingly ill on my treatment, were not supported by their answers to the questionnaire which patients are required to fill in before each consultation. On these a substantial improvement had been noted. When my lawyer enquired as to the reason for these discrepancies, their answer was that they did not wish to disappoint me.

Certainly, patients like these, would not make it possible for me to see the "100 patients per month during three days in Cape Town", as claimed in The Cape Metro.

Four years later, when E O'D presented her evidence at the Council hearing, she alleged that I had "provided empty lipstick cases to each of my patients, so that they could hide away the serum to the Belgium laboratory".

Emanating from the same two women, an article was published in 1996 claiming that I practised appendicectomies on patients as a means of treatment to cure them.

Through years of medical practice, I have learnt to recognise this rather odd category of patients who make it a point not to respond to treatment. They consider their disease as a trophy, pathologically so exceptional that nobody is bright enough to detect its existence or understand the mechanism. Therefore, no one will ever be capable of stripping them of it.

Regarding the matter of advertising, the charge accused me of "advertising with a view to professional gain" by "delivering, distributing, circularising, sent or published ... document, article or pamphlet". Advertising on the street corner, surmised the prosecutor in search of confirmation. The offending document transpired to be nothing but a list of recommendations, which are distributed to all patients before treatment. It advises them not to take the medication on an empty stomach, so as to avoid ulcers of the oesophagus or stomach. It warns them about skin becoming sensitive to the sun when taking tetracyclines. Also that they should not become dehydrated, or intoxicated, or pregnant, etc...

The fact that I had sent specimens overseas to my father rather than used the laboratories here in South Africa was always in the background, and obviously rankled. Could this be the reason that provoked them into confining a whole committee of respectable people for such a long period? Why did they not talk to me before opening fire?

When my lawyers asked them that question at the opening of the hearing, the answer was that they "did not know how to contact Dr Jadin at that stage" (Dr W).

After reading the newspapers, I was troubled for my

children. What would the reaction of their friends at school be the next morning?

My husband was distressed and, though he always supported me, my lawyers advised him it would be prudent to establish a clear distance between his practice and mine.

Indeed there was a chance that I might lose my medical registration with the South African Medical Council. My lawyers were convinced that I would receive some sort of sanction, and appeared to have been swayed towards the conclusion that my conduct was questionable.

Even though I could not comprehend the full context of the charge sheet, I knew I had done no wrong. Nevertheless, my confident nature did not seem to reassure them about the outcome.

As far as I was concerned, the story was a pack of lies, which could easily be refuted. I could not understand how such trumped up charges could come from medical colleagues. Could it be that they were upset by the immunological test used, or the success of my treatment?

The alarmed faces of my two advocates were my first serious shock.

This funny story was actually a sombre matter.

So, I started to collect and study mountains of medical books and scientific articles. Firstly, those on rickettsial infections, which were widely accepted regarding their symptomatology, diagnosis and treatment. I could find these in the French literature from the early Fifties until the mid Eighties originally, and then in the French, American and English literature from the beginning of the Nineties.

I also gave thorough consideration to the newly described Chronic Fatigue Syndrome (CFS). Criteria for this disease depended mainly on symptoms strictly defined by the Centre for Disease Control in Atlanta. Its aetiology was uncertain and the treatment very vague.

I fully investigated papers comparing different tests available for rickettsial infections. This revealed that the majority of them were in favour of the Micro-agglutination test, the test used by my father, as long as the antigens used were of good quality. The main concern expressed was about the skill of the laboratory technicians and the fact that the antigens were not available commercially. This was not the case in the alternative, the Weil-Felix test; it had been discredited for one reason or another by many authors, as I have explained before, when I discussed Pauline's diagnostic attempt. It is interesting to note that this test, up until the advent of Immunofluorescence and PCR, was the sole test approved by the SA Medical Board. It is also amazing to observe that the PCR test has already failed on reliability.

I discovered later that the same restriction to the Weil Felix test is widespread in many other countries.

I hoped that collecting and reading all these articles

would enable me to answer as scientifically as possible most of the questions likely to ensue. I also added my two attempts at publishing articles. I was feeling very well equipped and confident.

I had in my possession an affidavit written by a well-known South African psychiatrist. This doctor had been suffering from severe fatigue accompanied by muscle pain and depression, shortly after moving to a splendid farm in the heart of Natal. This place benefits from a generous rainfall, grazing is plentiful and the milk of the cattle herd is well known for its invigorating quality, if consumed before pasteurisation. Of course, those cows are hosts to ticks, which are themselves carriers of rickettsiae, parasites and other viruses. It is no secret that milk will remain contaminated if not heated sufficiently.

Seen from the plane, those hills of Natal are harmonious and green. Between two clouds, they appear to be interlaced by impressive rivers that often have difficulty following their course. The climate is definitely violent.

During one of my monthly visits to Pietermaritzburg, one of the most important towns in KwaZulu-Natal, I heard that the significant gorge seen just before the airstrip starts is called 'sleepy hollow'. Strange coincidence to give a name of legend to a place where ticks prevail.

This doctor had heard of my treatment and became my patient, as did his wife. Both of them were spectacularly cured. He resumed his duties and before retiring to his farm, treated 300 tired, depressed patients with the same treatment and the same success. He wrote a very elegant and perfectly detailed official report.

Besides this affidavit, I soon received a few hundred others send by happy recovered patients. I also received a batch of articles from a microbiologist in Melbourne, Australia, who, probably through my Australian patients, had come in contact with my father to whom he sent samples to be tested for rickettsia. My father had mailed him some French literature written by the Pastorian School during the late 80s, which he forwarded on to me. What was a great help was that he translated them into English.

So I was feeling safe and secure in my logical approach, my down-to-earth philosophy, my father's advice, my patients' health and support, and was blissfully unaware of my lack of understanding of the charge sheet.

The backbone of the charges were letters written by South African practitioners to the Medical Council and to each other.

I wish I were able to write this, as an author embarking on a novel would, so that my story need have no connection with reality, and the characters I describe should not exist in real life but belong to an imaginary world or dreamland.

However, since this is not exactly a novel, I will make

mention here of a few of them.

A physician from Durban whom I did not know, but who had plenty to say against me, reassuring one of his friends, wrote in this letter:

"Furthermore, a complaint about the treatment for a non-specified condition can only come from an aggrieved patient themselves, and not from a third party. One way or another, the whole treatment fiasco will die a natural death".

I recently saw one of his CFS patients whom he had treated for rickettsial infection with tetracyclines. He had only omitted to test him for this condition.

A medical doctor well known as a radio speaker, referring to me, declared: "Dr Jardin's activities must stop immediately". He also wrote a letter to the ME Association: "I agree that the activities of Dr Jardin are totally unacceptable. I recommend that you urgently contact 1) the Medicines Control Council and 2) the South African Medical and Dental Council, both in Pretoria". Signed by the Professor of the University of the W, on 17 March 1993.

Dr IW was working for the Institute of X, in the Immunology Department. She routinely carried out the Weil-Felix test for rickettsia. She published a paper in the March issue of the SAIMR newsletter (p.276) in 1992, with the intention of creating awareness amongst the medical fraternity about the misleading results given by the Micro-agglutination test done by my father.

She submitted her findings to laboratories and doctors and sent a copy of it to PA, director producer of a television program called 50/50, on 20 March 1992.

In this paper she presented data on supposedly three different sera tested for rickettsial infection, exhibiting the results of three different laboratories: the first, the Centre for Disease Control (CDC) in Atlanta, the second, the laboratory she was working for, and the third one emanating from my father's lab. She explained that the first two laboratories, Atlanta CDC and the SAIMR used the same technique, the Immunofluorescence test, and my father the Micro-agglutination test.

To enable her to succeed in her investigation, she wrote to some of my patients, asking them to donate their serum for analysis.

Three tubes were analysed to represent the conclusion of her statistics; she eventually admitted that she was "not quite sure anymore if there were three, but that two of them were taken from the same patient".

She solved the problem of her lack of antigens of Rickettsia prowazeki for the performance of the test, by writing in her publication: 'ND'. This stands for 'not done'.

She omitted to contact this "laboratory in Belgium that we have never heard of".

Without taking into consideration these points to establish the accuracy of the South African Institute for

Medical Research, she concluded: "As can be seen from the table, the results obtained by the SAIMR laboratory are in agreement with those of the CDC reference laboratory, while considerable differences are seen in the results reported by the Belgian laboratory. What can positively be said, however, is that the report of the CDC Rickettsial Reference Laboratory supports the accuracy of the SAIMR results."

It was getting too hot in this assembly; a storm had to explode.

Are you scared of storms?

Of storms? You must be teasing. We are concerned about the judgment of your mind, that allows you "to plead not guilty after treating patients in an unjustifiable and unscientific way, rendering potentially dangerous and medically unwarranted treatment, exploiting patients medically and financially, and touting, soliciting or advertising for patients" (Sunday Times, 25 August 1996).

Really? I will have to leave. The storm is there and I am even more scared of storms than stairs.

While you are hiding under the Medical Council's desk, we go out and look for patients who will listen to us and will complain about your treatment.

Well, anything is possible. Even that I would become paranoid.

The Executive Director of the ME Association was

determined to stop me. He compiled a mailing list to inform his members and subscribers about: "Rickettsia ... the Facts:

- There is no such illness called rickettsia.
- Blood tests done by the overseas lab are very primitive and unreliable.
- Tested positives there proved negative in different labs in South Africa. (NIV, University of Natal, various Labs & Bacteriologists UK)
- The doctor responsible for overseas tests and treatment understands very little about ME/CFIDS.
- People claiming recovery are misdiagnosed ME CFIDS.
- People claiming recovery are misdiagnosed or in remission ... for the time being."

This was published in the Myalgic Encephalomyelitis South African NEWS of March 1992, No 1.

At the same time, he sent a letter to Dr AS, complaining about this "very sad and grossly negligent situation".

In April 1992, he wrote to the Medical Association of South Africa "to protect sufferers and their families from exploitation... We established that both the Belgium testing and treatment regime were a rip off. What we do have here is, in our opinion, unethical practice, involving 'bogus' blood tests justifying 'experimental' treatment... We will continue to advise all to reject her claims and treatments...".

Left in ignorance, I only read this in 1996.

The same happened about an article entitled: Tetracycline in ME, fad or fact? written by BS and published by the South African Medical Journal (SAMJ) in July 1992.

In her "following list, not exhaustive, but serving to highlight a few of the dangers associated with tetracycline use in ME", she said that "in Canada a 16-year-old boy developed hepatic and renal failure a month after taking minocycline 10mg three times a day. The boy received a liver transplant. In addition, the patient had skin desquamation…" Frightening. But what is missing is the link connecting the child's illness and death, to my treatment methodology. It was not pointed out as a problem to consider. Perhaps no one realised the disparity in the cases described since doctors, having little time to read, only recognise the subject matter of the article from the title, and the warning of intra-cranial bleeding and permanent vision impairment. To highlight the danger, vitamin A was mentioned as part of the treatment, the very vitamin I emphasise should not be taken on my 'Do and Do Not' instructions, which are issued to all my patients.

The next paragraph of this article was about teratogenicity. It could of course devastate pregnant women. A check would have shown that I always make sure that I never treat pregnant women with tetracyclines.

The danger of "driving a vehicle during therapy", for example when patients are taking a specific kind of tetracycline such as minocyclin, was also debated in this article.

If there had been room for doubt concerning the perils of my treatment, it was underlined by her conclusion: "the familiar medical aphorism coined by Hippocrates, 'primum not nocere' (first of all, do not harm), embodies the need to discourage the injudicious use of expensive and potentially harmful drugs in ME sufferers. Although one should always remain open-minded about new theories and welcome original ideas regarding the pathogenesis and management of diseases, it is important to press for sound clinical studies before allowing anecdotes to mislead, potentially harm, and sometimes exploit an often vulnerable and desperate population."

An article in the Cape Metro soon followed the one in the SAMJ, specifying that: "Cape doctors said that in the light of the SAMJ's article and reports about Dr Jadin's work, they would not refer patients to her".

During the preparation of the case, a South African surgeon of French origin, Dr S, was appointed by the Council to translate some of my father's literature and that of other French scientists. He expressed his amazement to my lawyers: "Why should there be a court case for this?" He could clearly see that there was a scientific basis to my treatment.

However, much more was to come to reassure my guardian angels, particularly from the senior advocate, Mr JS, a well-spoken and well-reputed man. He did not miss a single opportunity to make my life miserable. I understand now that it was a question of technique, similar to the way a young horse is fenced in the warming arena, just before jumping in a competition. The young lawyer, SF, seemed to believe in my theory and practice, and put all his energy and intelligence into my defence.

At the third hearing, I realised that another member of the committee, Dr DJM, was also a colleague of the accusers, at the Institute. His attitude appeared quite neutral, but he was obviously not there by accident. So, on my lawyers' request, he was replaced.

I declined my lawyer's offer to use a translator, as well as so called experts in the subject. Indeed, who would I find in South Africa having expertise in a field, when the first step in the investigation, the validity of the Micro-agglutination test or even the Immunofluorescence test, was not available?

I thought about bringing in my father, should the situation worsen.

The session continued with three intelligent, sharp, discerning gentlemen on the panel: Prof FJM, Prof AF and Prof LAH.

When a member of the opposition referred to my case as a 'crusade', Prof FJM suggested that 'vendetta' would be more appropriate.

For day after day, they all listened quietly to the lies

delivered under the silent oath.

The members of the Institute of X feigned ignorance of my father's work. They vaguely pretended to have checked that he was still living in Belgium, but brushed off any knowledge of his work and did not believe that he still had a laboratory there. It was with pleasure that I showed the Committee a book titled Horizons 80 consisting of about 100 letters coming from all over the world and which was published to honour my father on the occasion of his 80th birthday.

With a little tremor in my voice, I read, as I was requested to, a letter from Prof Gear, dated August 1986, from the South African Institute for Medical Research:

Dear Professor Jadin

We understand that you will soon pass an important milestone in your life, the 80th anniversary of your birthday. So to begin, we wish you a very Happy Return of the day.

We first met in South Africa during World War II, and again in Leopoldville and Brazzaville at the ... Conference on Rickettsial Diseases in which you took a leading part. We heard about the red fever of the Congo and savannah typhus, as well as about rickettsial and chlamydial diseases. It was clear that you were making fundamental contributions to our knowledge of tropical diseases and have continued to do so ever since.

It is my privilege to express, on behalf of my South

African friends, our gratitude for a lifetime in the service of mankind, devoted especially to the welfare of the peoples who live in tropical Africa.

We salute you, one of the pioneers of tropical medicine in this century...

With appreciation and admiration,

Yours sincerely

James Gear

Dr IW, who, as mentioned earlier, had joined the opposition from the first days, managed for a few days to defend the impossible thesis she had previously published against me in the South African Medical Journal.

A general practitioner from Cradock, Dr D, travelled more than 1 000 km to complain about my rudeness towards him. Indeed, he wrote me a letter dated 20 December 1991, showing his interest in my work and saying how amazed he was by the "dramatic improvement" of one of his patients who I was treating. On the 24th of the same month and the same year, he wrote to the Medical Council complaining about me, not only for exploiting patients, but also for being such a rude person who had not answered his several letters.

Dr G, specialist in pharmacy, was appointed by the opposition as an expert to scientifically debunk my treatment and to confirm its harmful effect.

I am still puzzled at the way he used his powerful position.

He declared that he did not view CFS as a serious condition.

He condemned the dosages I was using as "four times too high", rather than criticising the duration of the treatment, and in the very next assertion contradicted himself and said that "where use in long term is when we develop the problems".

He refuted any reference supporting my "irrational treatment". First he rejected the Mims, a monthly publication updating the list, dosage and secondary effects of drugs available on the South African market. Because, according to him, "the information you have in Mims is what is inserted on the package, which may be registered 20 years ago". He then condemned the use of the Goodman and Gillman, in The Pharmalogical Basis of Therapeutics in my particular case, because it only "refers to tetracycline in general".

When my lawyer showed him a publication of a French scientist about the treatment of Q fever, he said he knew "French medicine very well" and said, "will not be impressed".

He concluded: "Mr Chairman, we cannot look at hundreds of funny little publications that somebody can bring up to substantiate what is not acceptable practice in antibiotic therapy in this country." The "somebody" was me and my scientific references were the "funny little publications" in the declaration under oath of Prof Dr G.

Prof T flew from the University of Cape Town to

support this accusation: I was "bizarre" and "therefore, some legal action should be taken against Dr Jadin". The fact that he had never seen me, nor spoken to me, did not seem to affect his serene confidence.

But, despite all this, a man, outstanding in his sense of curiosity and truth, supported me: Dr LVR. Even before I knew that there would be a case, he stood at my side, not passively, not by accident, but because of his belief in the truth of my approach.

He was, and still is, the director of an important group of pathological laboratories. He came to see my lawyers and me, a few days before the start of the hearing, to offer his help. As he had heard about the controversy over the Micro agglutination test, he himself went to visit my father in Antwerp, at the end of 1991, and testified in front of the Committee as to how impressed he had been by my father's knowledge, and by his laboratory. He explained that the lack of facilities and finances were the real restriction for the Micro agglutination test being used in a modern laboratory. He also outlined the fact that to keep the pool of antigens necessary to perform the test, there was a need to have animals, like guinea pigs or hamsters, which are no longer in use in South Africa for these purposes. He expressed his regrets at not having been able to communicate better with my father, due to the language barrier, and also wished to collaborate in the future with my father and me, concerning the antigens.

Some patients, or allegedly so, were called to testify against me.

Amongst them, one woman confirmed what she had previously reported to the newspapers: she saw me removing appendices in my Cape Town consulting room. To date, she added, I had removed about 50 appendices, brutally and on my own in my office. "Not in your sleep? Not when you were drunk?" later joked my lawyer.

The last patient to appear changed his mind when he understood that the questions he would have to answer could shake his integrity. He refused to be cross-examined.

The hearts of these patients were not beating at the same rhythm as the ones that later came to testify for me.

Amongst them there was my dear professor of ecology of the Witwaterstrand University, who could not help but give a brilliant lecture about scientific research, which left every one amazed.

An engineer thanked me for giving him his wife back after 15 years of disease.

Then too, there were the parents of my young patient whose future would have been to live in a mental institution, if it were not for my treatment.

Also came a lawyer, daughter of an eminent physician in Johannesburg, for whom the long debilitating illness had ended with the tetracycline treatment. There were numerous others with clear minds and grateful words.

A pharmacist was called from Port Elizabeth to testify against me, and my so-called deadly dosages of antibiotics. He was not quite sure how to answer the somewhat obscure questions put to him by the prosecutor, and after trying rather ineffectively, he eventually decided to cut a long story short and spoke without being asked about the noticeable improvement of my patients' condition since treatment. Suddenly, he was removed from the witness stand.

The assembly then adjourned and was rescheduled for a few months later.

Now, it was to be my turn to answer the various questions.

The work with the advocates intensified and there was no longer time to return home at night.

I shall remember until my dying day the last meeting before the hearing, early on a Sunday morning. The lift which was supposed to bring me from the parking lot to the lawyer's office on the tenth floor, was out of order: an electrical breakdown. With uncontrollable fear, I started the long ascent of those thousands of stairs in the dark, carrying what felt like a ton of documents containing accusations and evidence, and at each floor expecting to be assaulted by a robber. It was before the portable phone mania and I reached the office late and short of breath. As though to plunge me even further into despair, the Sunday Times was openly displayed at a page where they had published some more horror stories about me, coincidentally on 16 August, the day before the opening of my first week of self-defence. Looking up, two funereal faces welcomed me, and through the large windows, a winter sun rose.

This day had no end.

I was becoming tired of repeating the same stories to identical questions, always presented differently by my lawyers, for the purpose of developing the accuracy of my defence.

Then the advocate polished his technique: he went to fetch a fancy chair, designed by himself, to mimic the real witness box that I would have to enter the following day. He continued his cross-examination, as if at the theatre, when the final rehearsal takes place before the curtains are lifted for the first time.

He was sitting next to me. I was not allowed to look at him when he was asking his vicious questions. I had to speak facing an imaginary chairman. Suddenly, irritated by my hesitancy and my lack of witness skills, he exploded: "Look, since you are French, be more extrovert, speak to them, convince them, look them in the eyes, put your heart into it!" I was staring at the night falling on the skyscrapers of Pretoria, and shed tears for my destiny and my exhaustion. The young lawyer came to my rescue, and with some humour asked his colleague if he wanted a whip.

Of course, I do not blame them. They were professional and brilliant. They were applying rigorous principles to win the case, as the future would show.

After this incredible day, I was dropped off at a nearby guesthouse for the night; with the exhortation to study the 300 pages which we had not had time to read through together. It was midnight. I spent that night in a huge bed, screening my literature with the help of a few hi-lighter pens. They were pink, yellow, green, and my bed sheets were soon spotted the same way.

The next morning, I had to take my place on the witness stand. This consisted of a box almost two meters high resembling something from the Middle Ages. I was required to stand there for approximately one week. As I could not naturally reach the eyes of the auditorium, I bought a pair of incredibly high-heeled shoes. I was able to wear them only once more and that was in January 1997, the day of the verdict.

I was required to answer questions put to me by the prosecuting Council representing my adversaries. Although they sounded easier than those put by my lawyers, I was not prepared for the different approach. Moving incessantly from foot to foot, and with amazing speed and eloquence, he showered me with words. Using that obscure and tenacious technique, he resisted any attempt on my part for enlightenment. It was like a never-ending race, a parallelism being that of the logistic piece of work by Lewis Carroll, *Achille and the Tortoise*. He was being the hare, the calling one, and I was forced to be the tortoise, the consenting one. But

I did consent to each piece of evidence by adding a condition to it, which allowed the game to go on forever. Very often, he had suggested the condition I would use to restrict him.

He affected an approach guaranteeing that he would uncover the truth, but he was in fact burying it under a mountain of verbiage.

I suppose this is how students of law are trained to become prosecutors: confuse with words, appear to know all the answers and then convince with arguments.

I have never been involved in any sort of dialogue, which lasted as long and came to so little conclusion.

The prosecutor was in fact quite kind, and was too intelligent not to realise that he did not have a convincing case.

One day, he asked me why I treated a young girl, 14 years of age. The child recovered totally and the parents expressed the warmest appreciation in a thankful letter that then became part of the evidence. Therefore, I did not realise the point of the question at this stage. I obviously showed perplexity on my face. He appeared to wish to help me out by asking: "You mean, the proof of the pudding is in the eating?" After a short pause, while I reflected on the implication of this proverb, recognising Pauline's words, I agreed. The next morning, he questioned me on a similar letter from parents of another child recovering as a result of my treatment. Once again not realising that I was not supposed to treat children with tetracyclines, I was quick with my answer: "The proof is in the pudding." At this misquotation, a ripple of laughter ran through the assembled audience.

The only time I lost my cool was when the prosecutor accused me of taking advantage of a free air ticket to Cape Town, Pietermaritzburg and Port Elizabeth. I must explain here how this came about. Patients at these centres had got together and devised a plan whereby instead of all independently making a trip to Johannesburg for their checkups, they would club together and pay my fare to enable me to see them in their hometowns. I accepted this offer innocently, before I appreciated what these types of trips are all about — meaning having to endure the plane's fridge-like atmosphere, the tiredness of long hours' work and the night drives back home through Johannesburg, the aggressive city.

Later, in this frame of mind, I painted a canvas. The subject was a sky, seen from an aeroplane with puffy, V-shaped clouds, which had something in common with a SOS. My intention was to give it to the prosecutor, but I forgot and it still hangs in my waiting room, like a bitter reminder.

While we were closeted in the auditorium, arguing all those heavy charges against me, the secretary's office of the Medical Council had been inundated with hundreds of faxes from my patients, praising my work and me. The view expressed by those reams of paper should have stopped the session in its tracks. But the ritual was not so democratic.

Then came January 1997.

After almost two years of stress, spent studying how best to defend my theory and myself in public, and how to lecture on the subject of rickettsia and CFS, my tongue had dramatically improved its English pronunciation, and my synapses had been enhanced and sharpened by stimuli directed at me by the examining Committee. Unexpectedly the Committee announced an end to this procedure. When they asked me if I was not feeling too offended by the modus operandi, I comforted them and thanked the assembly for improving my knowledge of their language and my understanding of medicine.

Before the last hearing, with a sense of absurdity, which probably protected me from fainting, I asked my lawyers how I would be executed: guillotine, electric chair, hemlock? They did not recognise my irony or found it inappropriate, since they answered me seriously: "no death penalty, no jail sentence". Certainly, I had not killed or damaged anybody but "probably a suspension of practicing medicine. Maybe three years…" But most probably I would have to stop my treatment forever. I was dismayed.

Eventually the afternoon of Friday, 17 January 1997 arrived when, in front of a tense public, the chairman of this Committee announced its decision. The majority of the people present were my patients. The media was also there. Dr AS, the convenor of my detractors, was sitting next to a mountainous woman, both of them wearing dark glasses and constantly whispering to each other. Not to mention my presence and my frozen eyes like a sheep staring at a wolf. My lawyers, also present, did not look very relaxing either.

The Chairman went through each charge on the list of accusations, one at a time, but not in any specific order.

A cat playing with a mouse.

He acquitted me of all charges, finishing with these words: "Although the committee has found Dr Jadin not guilty on all the charges brought against her, the committee wishes to make the following comments and recommendations with regard to her practice:

"In the absence of any evidence as to the reliability or not of Prof Jadin's Micro-agglutination test, and in view of the disquiet expressed by the committee concerning this investigation, it is recommended that there be a proper evaluation of the Micro-agglutination test against the Immunofluorescence test (IGM and IGG) with all important rickettsial strains.

"That the results of this evaluation and the clinical results of your therapy be published in a scientific journal, perhaps with the assistance of one of the members of the Medical Schools."

Heat waves of the end of January in South Africa had evaporated the tension of the situation, as would the fumes of a Turkish bath.

After five years of uncertainty, I was relieved and most impressed by the impartiality of these three judges, and the courage it required to find me innocent of a host of accusations lodged by their own colleagues.

I subsequently kissed them, as well as my relieved lawyers, said goodbye and went home carrying files and flowers.

The following day, still shaking, I resumed my work.

In its next edition, the Sunday Times continued its retaliation with the following headline: 'Yuppie flu doctor let off the hook'.

(19th of January 1997, by Cas St Leger.)

Then, still in bold but a smaller print, she wrote: "A controversial yuppie flu expert charged with disgraceful conduct was advised this week to modify her treatment, which some experts have warned is dangerous" and sustained to the end of the article "anger, despair and helpless feelings".

After this long experience, I had still expected the newspapers to report the truth.

However, despite this tabloid discredit, the number of my patients exploded.

Without the complaints of my colleagues, I would never have intensified my studies. Without their unintentional publicity, I would never have so rapidly reached this number of patients. That court case was the vital key to my success.

As a result of this uncalled-for torture, I slid a foothold into the scientific world and kept the other anchored in the clinical practice, so that I could step from one to the other to better advance. This is a big advantage over other scientists, for example, clinicians describing diseases without access to their causative agents, or pathologists explaining germs' cycles before placing them in their main interesting container: humanity.

A few months later, in 1998, the University of Newcastle invited me to my first conference at the International Congress on CFS in Manly, Sydney, Australia.

Shortly after my arrival, a dear friend and her husband took me in. Thanks to them, I fell in love with life in Sydney, where I returned the next year to present my work at the same congress on CFS.

In September 1999, I had the opportunity to expose my latest developments at a congress in Brussels, Belgium, and during a conference at the beautiful University of Padoua, Italy.

Each of those trips gave me the chance to meet and discuss with the world leaders of CFS. Besides Philippe Bottero, a family friend that became a personal friend, and also one of the real pioneers in treating rickettsial diseases, there was the enthusiastic and impressive Tim Roberts from the University of Newcastle, and his team, the Belgian Kenny De Meirleir from the Vrye Universiteit of Brussels, the American Garth Nicolson from the Institute for Molecular Medicine of USA, WJ Martin from the centre of Complex Infectious Diseases of USA, Dan Peterson from the George Washington University School of Public Health, and last but not least Vincento Cutrupti from Italy.

Enough time has now elapsed to summarise my 'after investigation' duties.

I have contacted every laboratory in every town of South Africa about the Immunofluorescence test, so as to carry out a comparative study with the Micro-agglutination test of Giroud.

No success.

Up until now, only the Weil Felix test appears on the entire laboratory test request forms with the word 'rickettsia' in the result column.

Since early in 2000, three types of chlamydia and one type of mycoplasma antibodies have become available, to increase the serological investigations I am doing.

Recently, Coxiella burnetti antibodies have also become obtainable. Just like chlamydia and mycoplasma, it has been isolated as it is a specific group.

Valuable help comes from various independent laboratories that serologically confirm my diagnoses.

One day, I shared with Dr LVR my anxiety about the comparative study between the two serological tests, which I had to perform to satisfy the Medical Council. He confessed that the IFA test was not routinely performed and advised me to contact the SAIMR, where I might be lucky.

My quest was in vain.

I then wrote a letter addressed to the Medical Council explaining why I was not able to accomplish this impossible mission.

CHAPTER 6:

WHAT RESEARCH TAUGHT ME

"Scientific research has the following point in common with love stories: they would not be looked for if one would know before hand how time will treat them."
—Jean Rostand—

The court case forced me to study in depth the relationship between rickettsia and CFS.

All the information I gathered was more captivating than I could ever have imagined. I learnt not only about other infectious diseases, but also about other fields of medicine like immunology, haematology, pharmacology, cardiology, rheumatology and endocrinology.

I realised that fascinating studies are pursued with success in various research centres in the world. They often represent a step forward in the treatment of diseases, but repeatedly those studies are dropped and forgotten for different reasons.

Nobody will gather the precious conclusions. The research team is dissolved with no survivor.

The ideas were disposable ones.

Contrary to the pastorian school, they belong rather to the food industry, with a present purpose to fulfil. When their mission is achieved, they dissolve, looking for the next function. Since they were not building with either vertical or horizontal structures, their destiny is to collapse.

And in another country, in another language, the same study is going the same way, with the same success and will fade away.

The two schools rarely cross paths. Perhaps they do not speak the same language or they do not practise the same religion. Maybe their political alliance is different, or is it only a question of technical experience? Such is the case with the 500 publications of my father, in French, most of which are lost to the English scientists.

Those factors jeopardise medical evolution and leave us wandering in our discipline like the builders of the Tower of Babel, without geographical and historical perception.

In the meanwhile, patients are looking for solutions to their troubles.

If this is not given by the medical world, they will

logically explore parallel or alternative medicines. The success that they will meet in the procedure will quantify the development of those disciplines.

Charlatans as well as honest scientists are available.

Due to the lack of any legislation in those new fields of healing arts, they will be, more than anywhere else, difficult to distinguish.

As a child, modern medicine looked pretty perfect to me. Top technology opened doors for us. No stone was left unturned and everything had an approved explanation.

University did not really change those beliefs of mine. We had to assimilate the first year before moving to the second. One subject followed another with an implacable logic.

After seven years of successful studies, I qualified as a medical doctor from the University of Louvain, Belgium, considered an excellent medical school in Europe.

It took me years to realise that medicine is not more logical than the human being. Medicine is a human grasp of diseases and like the sea approaching the beach, a wave will follow a wave, untiringly, using the same water over and over, following guidance that is beyond our control and our comprehension.

We belong to a world not manageable by our reason. And the only way to cross it is to join the irrationality.

Indeed, a man convinced that after him nothing will remain of what he has done, can only become disillusioned and stop his productivity. He will go on strike against creation. Nevertheless, to go on strike against creation, is to go on strike against himself.

And the irrationality will take over if he decides to keep his human status, as Jean Rostand observed.

Again, he has to get lost so that he can find himself once more.

I do not have the philosophical ingenuity and the courage of Socrates. Instead of choosing the hemlock, I innocently dream of a scientific world where the waste of energy due to the lack of communication will finally be stopped.

Where, for instance, the agent of trachoma discovered in the early 1950s, as quoted above, and the other chlamydia would be part of a routine diagnostic test, because of their epidemiological value.

Where the recurrent Malgache fever would be the starting point of the control of Lyme disease. Looking at its new name, this disease appears to emerge from America, which masks its worldwide distribution. Borders emerge instead of disappearing.

Why has the trail opened by Legag, Giroud, Jadin and many others about the pathology of neurological, cardiac and vascular diseases, still no access?

The modern scientist, proud of his new technology, forgets to look for short cuts to new discoveries in the tracks of his predecessors. He is convinced that the rigorous application of techniques is the only up-to-date value of reaching a medical diagnosis.

Germs causing diseases belong to the living world, not to the static world.

When technology describes life, it comes with the perfect picture of a microbe, in other words its ID book, with its own and unique prints.

Unfortunately, the live world never stops metamorphosing.

This is why the mutation taking place while the experts are concentrating on their work, is omitted.

Therefore technology can only approach the successions of mutations of life, but is always at least one step behind.

While the period spent in never-ending discussions has ended, sick people, also called patients as if they needed to be convinced of a time factor, are waiting, recovering or dying.

Their doctors have gone to academic meetings, in search of refined technology to enable them to capture the present pathological entity, to define our revolving world.

When they come out, divided by conflicts to find harmony, it is already tomorrow for the germs, as well as for the patient — who have both had the opportunity to change shape in order to keep their power.

Except in Antarctica, where germs hibernate or die, this ugly crowd will never stop crumbling the cosmos and disintegrating it through its implacable kaleidoscopic pepper-grinder. Not seen, not known. Whites, blacks, and yellows will be crushed in a dark homogeneous dust. In panic or in unconsciousness.

The natural evolution of life escapes mathematics.

Of course 2+2 will stay 4, only if no mutation takes place.

But this is the foundation of life.

Life, no matter what we guess in our scientific mind, does not follow one road, but all the possible roads, and preferably the one where it will succeed. And our logical mind does not ponder on those roads.

In 1995, I met a South African microbiologist who had published a paper about the relationship between chlamydia and cardio-vascular diseases. He stressed that this study had nothing to do with rickettsia, which he knew nothing about, as, according to him, it did not exist in South Africa.

He showed me beautiful microscopic photographs of atheroma plaques, from which he had isolated chlamydia. First time it was ever demonstrated, he said proudly. He ignored, and was not interested in knowing, that in 1962 Guy Delanoe conducted similar research on rickettsia in the Cardiology Department of Casablanca, while Nicolau came to the same conclusions in Romania, as published on many occasions in the Bulletin de la Société de Pathologie Exotique in the early 1960s. In 1966, Griest published a microscopic picture of rickettsia in the coronary arteries of humans.

More recently, when I was in Italy, I heard discussions and read articles about the use of antibiotics in the treatment of myocardial infarct.

The incompatibility between French and English is well established, ever since the English burned Joanne of Arc at the stake, in Rouen. Or maybe this incompatibility is more fundamental. Is it not strange indeed for a Latin mind to gauge people and boats in feet, horses in hands, weight in stones, distance in miles, liquid in gallons and that the number ten becomes a dozen. At this point of perplexity, they add mint to improve the taste of both their meat and their chocolate.

But, what about the rivalry between the Italian and the Anglo Saxon world, which is much more radical and unheard of? Radical, because for many Italians, the English language is largely thought of as being painful to the ear, unheard of, because those same Italians avoid contact with the English world. Taking into consideration the perception that the world consists in North Italy, South Italy and Paris will stop any dispute developing. It is my experience that the modern Italian doctors are well trained in recognising rickettsial diseases.

On the other hand, Russian scientists carry a political burden, which directs their evolution in the whole world, but which also forces them to cultivate very specific strains of germs in their laboratories, and amongst them there are rickettsiae, as a biological weapon. My father, though, used his Russian connections as a diagnostic tool.

One could study the influence of politico-economic factors on the scientists and their research and this, together with the human thirst for power and fame, would give prominence to the hazardous progression of medicine.

Profitable researches are in daily danger.

Discoveries remain atomic in time and space, and so seldom grow to be molecules sustaining operational units, which would be in charge of building the future on the past, whatever the country of origin.

Here we are, at the beginning of a millennium, where communications are becoming so fluent that all those barriers, and their excuses, have not the same reasons to be.

Computerisation, by swallowing our universe, has not finished to shake its foundation.

Recent world conferences relating to different scientific subjects, as CFS and fibromyalgia, resemble a project on planetary medicine.

This concept probably appears more eccentric and pointless to certain scientists than the litigious discussion about the presence or the absence of rats infesting the city of London. But the powerful and disciplinary organisation ruling in an ant colony does not apply to the medical profession where individualism too often

gives the final answer. Nevertheless, the medical fraternity is not entirely dissenter, impenetrable to other
people's ideas, guided only by politics, glory or money,
and resisting to any technical progress.

Most of us are in friendly contact with other research
centres. At our disposal, we have fax lines and email. We
manage to take aeroplanes. We reveal our work, we
listen to other fellows, and, back home, we remember
what was said, sometimes.

There is nothing more natural to man than these
exchanges between scientists. Nothing to do with
metaphysics.

Is it not why he has ears, eyes, a mouth with a tongue,
a brain with a memory and not just a box, filled with
megabytes?

Surely, that is the advantage of his human nature.

The disadvantage of his physical shape clearly stands
in the way of the dispatching potential, which right
now, has to make use of a walk, a horse, a bike, a
sputnik, a plane or a ship. Whatever the choice, the trip
will be exhausting, often boring, always endless and
bursting with hazards — unpleasant and needless, if not
lethal.

The discovery of a fast way of transport, which will
bring the human being from one corner of the
universe to the other — just like a light electron, free
to live and die wherever, will be the end of the other
side of the world.

The achievement of this dream is only a derivative of

human mind, presenting the same raw material, but seen from a different angle.

We stay in our area.

It is more a new record to foresee than a dilemma to overcome

Afterwards, one will also have to reinvent fiction.

That will be more difficult.

So, medical sciences do not thrive better in the computer network than in the mathematical set-up. Not much to unveil with the severity of mathematics, even with the help of infallible statistics, and nothing for a skilled computer to decode.

Beyond its own mutation, it has to face unknown factors, constantly building up or down. As the darkness of Aladdin's thousand and one nights, will-o'-the-wisps appear and disappear without warning. How much chaos to overcome, and how many quick clear fires to avoid before defining a bit of science.

Medicine is always refutable. It describes general rules, which always need exceptions to be confirmed. As long as the exception is not found, its existence cannot be denied. And when found, there is still doubt about its exceptional nature.

This applies to every level of medical science. Let us take the example of a prognosis. What could be more self-doubting than a prognosis following a diagnosis, which in itself has a refutable foundation?

The only acceptable prognostic is the one described by Albert Dastre. "To say that a man is dead is only a prognosis". Because, in this case, the diagnosis is irrefutable.

In fact, medicine concurs much better with meteorology and should be expressed in the same language based on hypothetical percentages, to express its convictions.

What a trump to adapt continuously to an evolutive disease and abstain from giving a short-term forecast, even though the medical pedestal is eroded from the layman's view. For instance, our prognosis for today would be a 30 percent chance of flooding on the South Coast, and not this patient with leukaemia only has two months to live; or tomorrow morning, the sky will be cloudy, followed in the afternoon by sunshine and occasional storms and not, this depressed patient will be considered as such and treated with antidepressants for the rest of his life so that his complains will not change anymore.

There is no need to panic. The more the brain is convoluted and divided into deep fissures, the more easily the possibilities of generating an imbalance, which mixes thoughts and prompts new opinions. Lobotomy is based on this principle.

Subsequently, one just needs to organise ideas in an easily accessible area of the remaining cortex to improve the short-term memory of the owner. For the long-term memory, he will have to move information into a deeper fold of the brain.

Less precise than a stroke of the chisel looking for a face in a marble sculpture, less unexpected than a mixture of colour on a painter's palette, medicine is before anything an art, so fascinating and so deceptive.

This discipline is heavy in contingencies not mentioned in any books.

Actually, medicine is a newborn of the century, waiting for a more refined technology to be properly delivered.

To me, today's medicine is still as enigmatic as abstract art. As untouchable as a dolphin. As probable as the digit seven.

CHAPTER 7:

ABOUT RICKETTSIAE, PARA-RICKETTSIAE AND OTHER TICK-BORN DISEASES.

"To appreciate a thing,
You must first isolate it."
—*JK Chesterton*—

One must not count on the size of things.

The tick, as small as it looks, is a real biological bomb, carrying around a multitude of powerful micro-organisms. It has been written that some of those have already been used as such, and that others are isolated and kept for this intention.

It will take the female tick from 178 up to 275 days — depending mainly on temperature — to give birth to between 100 and 1 000 eggs. After this laying, life ends.

Nymphs have six legs and as soon as they are hatched, rush to perform their mission as killers. Heaving itself on any means given by nature, they wait for a host into which they can insidiously dig their claws. Directed by their instinct, they wait patiently in this world as vast as their despair. Because this world is too big, and they come from so far and they are exhausted. Eventually, a pitiful mouse stops on its way to quench its thirst. Our floor neighbour, the rat suspends its automatic path since it has found some peelings acridly perfumed. The forbidding hedgehog becomes, if necessary, an altruistic host with a flesh as delicious as the one of the sea urchin, and this bird, still pathologically innocent, will become a new messenger after having been used as a feeding platform. A motionless lizard waiting for a fly has enough blood, even though cold, to be transformed into the start stone of a new rickettsial dynasty.

Our planet is more inhabited than we think.

A few days later, larvae, heavy with their blood collection, fall on the ground and start a very productive digestion.

Their forms change: they now have eight legs for the next role, which is to suck again an Amphitryon, to fall again to the ground and to change into an adult tick or imago.

Inhabiting a world as a soldier of a Lilliputian army,

these forms are here to guarantee the kingdom of boredom does not settle in our Gulliver's bodies.

The boredom would make us worried, as would any human civilisation without threats — a civilisation structured, free of every dangerous animal and any adventurous condition.

There would be no fear.

No fear, except of death that we did not manage to avoid or store in a forgotten prehistoric gallery. It looks more sordid amidst this perfect organisation. One can see it coming so well. There is no obstacle to cross while waiting for it, we have too much leisure, too much time to ask questions. We need an antidote to this anachronism. Drugs.

Drugs to fill the boredom, introduced in full conscience, while the contingent of microbes land like a surprise. Their genius is similar to Hieronymus Bosch, Flemish painter of the sixteen century with this rich theme: the last judgement. With their bites they disintegrate our human condition into hybrids of hermetic beings.

Skin thickens, a male impregnates a female, randomly in the impromptu bridal layers of hair, feathers, and dust.

Three years go by.

It is the arrival line, which joins the start line.

In case of famine, larvae can survive for one year without food, nymphs for two years, and adult ticks have three years of storage time.

The nomadic life of these insects allows them to accumulate all sorts of infectious germs. During a walk, the tick carries along an unsuspected world of the infinitely simple, the infinitely minute, and the infinitely complementary. The assortment is corrosive and insidious. It is a long procession, which drifts through our human fable in silence.

Except for ticks, rickettsiae and para-rickettsiae use other numerous ways of transport, mainly public transport. There are not only small arthropods' bodies which put up with them, like fleas, mites and lice, but also amoeba from water and other protozoas.

A few decades ago, rickettsiae were consecutively considered as being viruses or bacteria. In fact they are neither. They belong to a group of intracellular germs with a poor enzymatic component. Therefore, they have to use for survival, the enzymatic system of the cell they invade. Energy produced by the Krebs cycle will do. Using the ribosome in the cytoplasm, they feed, grow and multiply by binary division.

Coxiella burnetti differs from other rickettsia in that it is enclosed in a vacuole during growth and division.

In in-vitro cultures, rickettsiae classically resemble short little sticks surrounded by a membrane. Different groups have different forms.

Among them, Rickettsia prowazeki is the only flagellated organism in this family.

In diluted buffered salt solutions, isolated rickettsiae

are unstable. They lose metabolic activity and infec-
tivity for animal and human cells. But if potassium,
sucrose and serum albumin are added, their survival is
considerably increased. Physicians treating patients
infected with rickettsia should remember those facts.

Rickettsial infection was discovered in 1909, when
Ricketts saw and described the germ that causes
Rocky Mountain Spotted Fever (RMSF) in man.
Ricketts, as well as another scientist, Prowazek,
contracted typhus and died.

Chlamydia and mycoplasma were classified under the
rickettsial group throughout the world, until a couple
of decades ago. This is still applied in the Russian books
of microbiology.

So, discrepancies about classification are related to the
different schools describing them at different times.

Mycoplasmas characterise themselves by the absence
of a typical cell wall during their entire life. They are
just contained in cytoplasmic membrane, which gives
them an allomorphic aspect. Being opportunistic
germs, dust is described as being their vector or
support. But this is far from being specific to that
species. Indeed, ticks and other arthropods release
faeces and eggs in the ground and they themselves, as
well as their products, will eventually be turned into
dust.

The species mainly described are Mycoplasma
hominis, Mycoplasma fermentis and Mycoplasma
pneumoniae. Their laboratory growth requires a rich

medium containing serum proteins and a sterol. They incorporate a concentration of up to 65% of cholesterol into the cell membrane. What is the clinical repercussion of this transfer?

Chlamydias were recently the subject of intensive studies in the USA, which gives a geographical reason for their declassification. They were described as an independent group because they do not need arthropods to be transmitted to man.

They are mostly contained in a vacuole inside the cytoplasm of the host's cell, where they multiply by repeated binary fission before being released after the rupture of the host's cell.

Amongst them, we find the Chlamydia trachomatis of Paul Giroud, the Chlamydia psittaci coming from South America's birds, the Chlamydia pneumoniae, all loading an atmosphere of menace for our lungs, heart, neurological and uro-genital system.

Even if rickettsial diseases have lost their leadership role in today's world, a rigid classification is hazardous. The differentiation of those very similar germs, which carry about the same pattern of action and have the same vector, will have no influence on their response to the same treatment.

Here are a few species names:
R. Prowazeki, R. Quintana, R. Rochalima, R. Mooseri, R. Africa, R. Australis, R. Conori, R. Rickettsii, R. Siberia,

R.Acari, R. Montana, R. Burnetti, R. Tsutsugamushi, R. Sennetsui, R. Canada, R. Orientalis, R. Bellii, R. Bedsonia, R. Sheila Smith, R. Malish, R,Wilmington, R. rhipicephali, R. Pisci, R.Texiana, R. japonica, R. Heilonlg –jiangi, Israeli tick typhus R., R. aeschlimannii, R. Helvetica, R. honei, R. japonica, R. massiliae, R. mongolotimonae, R. parkeri, R. slovaca, R. sp. A-167, R. sp Bar29, R. sp.BJ-90, R. sp. DaE100R, R. sp. DnS14, R. DnS28, R. FUJ98, R.HL93, R.HLJ-054, R. sp. IRS4, R. sp. IRS3, R.sp.RpA4, R. sp. S, R. cooleyi, R. felis, R. moreli, R. peacockii, R. sp.'Digas and Belikov 1999.', R. sp. 'La copita', R. sp. Midichlorii, R. sp. IrR/Munich, R. sp. MOAa, R. sp. PAR (pea aphid Rickettsia), R. sp.WB-8-2, male-killing R. from Adalia bipunctata, male-killing R. from Adalia decempunctata, papaya bunchy top disease R., R. amblyommii, R. bellii, Coxiella burnetti, etc...

To be virulent, germs sometimes have to form a partnership — to their advantage to improve their sketchy ability, and to the disadvantage of their host's immune system.

Alone, they will only cause a few temporary problems in their victims.

Of course, our defence system is not going to collapse at the first tremor.

The production of an antibody clone is usually easy. But complications arise when different antigenic aggressions are combined. It is therefore rare in consultation to see a patient suffering only from a unique infection.

It is not to add confusion that I advise to consider each medical case through a corrective prism: the same germ, or rather, the same association of germs can cause different diseases, and different germs can cause the same disease. This Arian's clew is always handy to keep when having to enter into the labyrinth of those striking pathologies.

So, Lyme disease has points in common with rickettsial diseases, since the vectors are the same, as are the symptoms and finally the treatment.

But, as discussed before, the agent is a spirochete, Borrelia burgdoferi, described in 1975, in Connecticut where a psychosis erupted, an apocalyptic tick panic. Local children were not allowed to frolic on the green grass but were amused on carpets of plastic lawn. Telephone companies provided Help lines 'SOS Lyme' 24 hrs a day in several states. Ticks in America are now regarded with terror and premonition — a medical emergency. And remarkably, the rest of the world is quite indifferent.

Once again, it is impossible to ignore Drury and its Borrelia duttoni when in the presence of recurrent fevers. Ticks transmit it and the illness looks like a rickettsial infection: chronic fatigue, associated with neurological and rheumatic symptoms. The cutaneous rash caused at the entry site of the parasite at the skin level, is called 'erythema migrans' which means 'fleeting redness' in Latin. Its appearance varies and can even look like the black spots seen in Rocky Mountain spotted fever or in Mediterranean spotted fever.

The erythema migrans as well as the 'black spot' and the tick bite are often not mentioned in the history of the disease.

Spirochetes Borrelia hermsii and Borrelia turicatae are the agents of tick-born relapsing fever. Small and soft ticks, the Ornithodoros, which only feed at night, transmit them. Like lots of ticks, they leave chemicals on the skin consisting of an anticoagulant and an analgesic, to confuse the issue. Another kindness of nature.

Apart from Lyme disease, rickettsiae and para-rickettsiae (chlamydia and mycoplasma), ticks can still cause many other infections. Among them, babesioses, caused by a protozoa, Piroplasma babesia microti, colonising the red cells, cause a disease very similar to malaria. It is found in association with rickettsial infections and Lyme disease and is very commonly found in splenectomised patients. Therefore, the disease will be severe and of long duration, and the treatment inefficient.

Erlichiosis, often considered as a rickettsiosis, is a parasite of humans, fish, canines and horses. In the latter, the disease manifests as an intestinal malabsorption. The germ penetrates the white cells and causes leucopoenia and a thrombocytopenia, as well as liver abnormalities. Erlichia platys of canine origin has just been described for the first time in Australia in early 2001. Coming from Africa, it was isolated in the US in 1978. Congratulations to those scientists looking in the cycle of this cousin of Erlichia rickettsii.

Colorado tick fever, also described in France and Belgium, is a viral disease caused by Coltovirus.

Another viral disease transmitted by ticks is Powassan encephalitis. The survivors will suffer from neurological symptoms irreversibly disturbing.

These two viral infections can be transmitted by blood transfusion.

Tularemia, for which the agent is Francisella tularensis, could be caused by a tick bite or direct skin contact with an infected animal. It is found in rabbit breeders and hunters. The disease starts with swollen glands, becoming abscesses, complicated by fistulae. These fistulae, sometimes appearing spontaneously, are more often a consequence of surgical investigations. Other symptoms include fever, headaches, abdominal pain and … fatigue.

Tick paralysis is the only disease ticks transmit without any vector, but directly via a neurotoxin produced in the salivary glands. That way, the victim may be paralysed, suffering from chronic muscle weakness or may even die.

Those infectious agents are various in number and morphology. Nevertheless the symptoms they display are very similar. Most of them are difficult to isolate in the lab. What a long tunnel we have to cross before reaching them.

It is not enough to play with the magnification lens of a microscope to identify the life crawling in our arteries. It would be so much easier if they expressed one face only, and if that face were printed via our retina on our brain, just like light would do on features or on body angles.

From here, the desk where I am writing, I contemplate the Indian Ocean, magnificent. As a man finishes his swim and surfaces inevitably, with no choice but to offer his naked shape to me, stealing his identity.

If this would apply to our pathological monsters, a good technician specialised in pure morphology would be consulted and would give us a diagnosis. It would be enough to see and to understand.

No. We have to observe alternately phenomena belonging to completely different fields. We have to add them, subtract them, to guess and then to ignore them. "To observe is the mysterious gift to see with the eyes," according to Mallarmé. A rare gift, often badly judged and mistaken for curiosity. Unfortunately this latter is often considered a fault and what is more, a female one in which nobody should indulge — and above all not a doctor.

But without curiosity, there is no observation.

Without observation, there is no link possible between discrepancies.

20 November 1986

Dear Professor Jadin

We understand that you will soon pass an important milestone in your life - the 80th anniversary of your birthday so to begin We wish you a very Happy Birthday and many Happy Returns of the Day.

We first met in South Africa during World War 2 and again in Leopoldville and Brazzaville at the WHO Conference on Rickettsial Diseases in which you took a leading part. We heard about the red fever of the Kongo and savannah typhus as well as about rickettsial and chlamydial diseases It was clear that you were making fundamental contributions to our knowledge of tropical diseases and have continued to do so ever since

It is my privilege to express on behalf of your South African friends our gratitude for a lifetime in the service of mankind devoted especially to the welfare of the peoples who live in tropical Africa

We salute you - one of the pioneers of Tropical Medicine in this century.

With appreciation and admiration
Yours sincerely
James Gear

One of the letters from the book Horizons 80,
written to my father who was approaching 80,
by Prof James Gear from the South African
Institute of Medical Research.

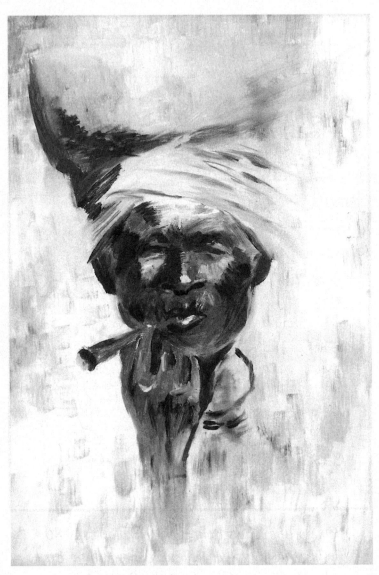

One of my paintings.

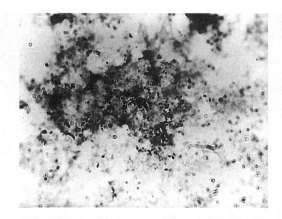

Slide showing a micro-agglutination test.

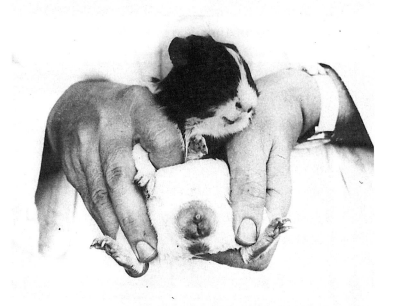

*A guinea pig with inflamed testis after being contami-
nated with a strain of rickettsia.*

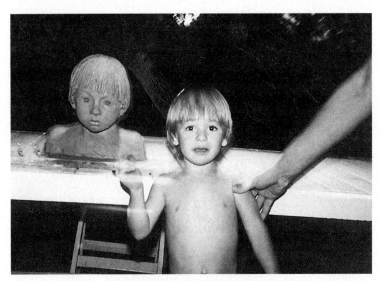

My son Antoine and his bust.

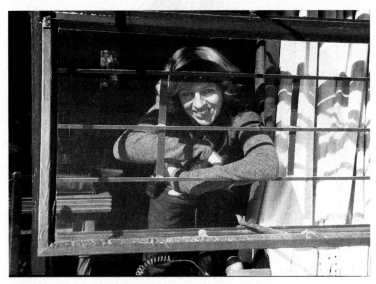

At home in Johannesburg

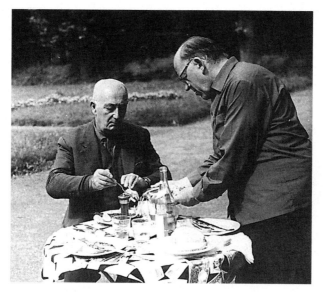

Paul Giroud (left) and Jean-Baptiste Jadin in Arbre.

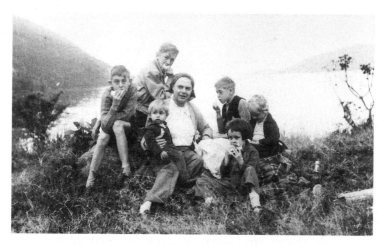

The Jadin family having a picnic along Lake Kivu.

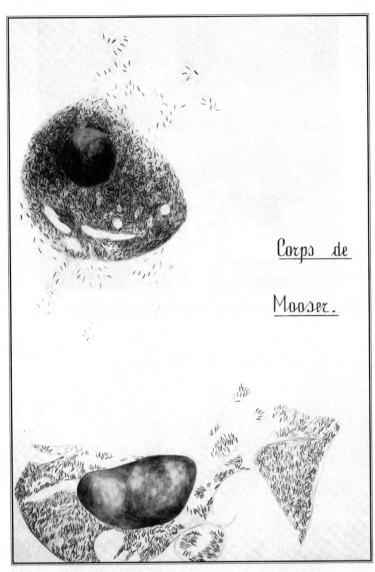

Corps de Mooser.

Mooseris' corpuscules (rickettsia) seen from a vaginal smear of a guinea pig.

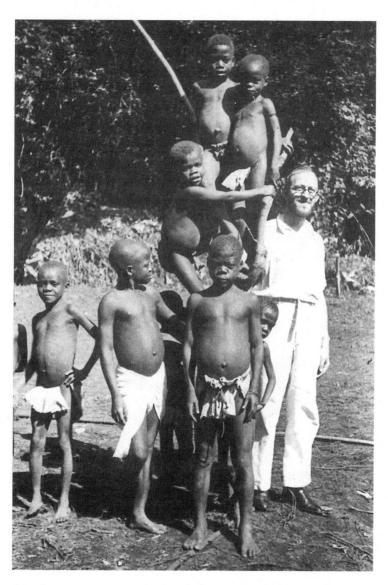

Dr Jean-Baptiste Jadin and the Pygmies in Ituri Forest.

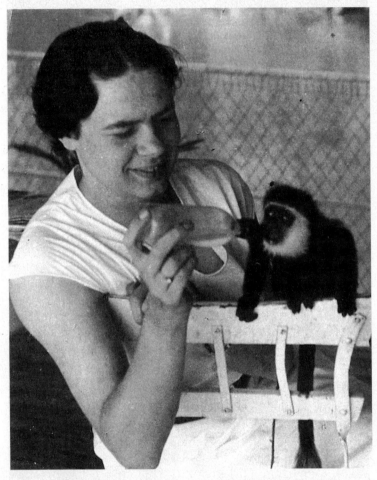

My mother and Colobe in the animal nursery.

With no link, where is the intelligence that allows us to understand our surroundings?

The world is tedious, even if limited to the tick and its little body. How many megabytes do we require to enable us to list its parasites?

Furthermore, without wanting to be pessimistic, this list is probably the visible part of the iceberg or, according to an African proverb, the ears of a hippopotamus nonchalantly soaking in the lake.

Moreover, any good and respectable logic will not associate a pair of dull and half closed eyes with the mass of cytoplasm confined in this submerged volume.

The world's appearance is not linked to its content.

CHAPTER 8:

TRANSMISSION OF INTRACELLULAR MICRO ORGANISMS

"It is not for the rose the bird lands on the rose tree:
it is because of the rose beetle."
—*Jules Renard*—

The tick has fascinated man for a long time. The first descriptions found date back to the remotest times.

During the first century AD, the Roman author Pliny wrote: "Ticks bury their heads in flesh to suck the blood from which they nourish themselves." He concluded: "The tick is the only animal that does not have an opening for faecal elimination, thus it dies as it is feeding, releasing its host when its becomes too heavy."

162

It is true that the tick drops after feeding, as it needs this fall, followed by its reattachment onto an animal, or a human, to attain its adult form. But it is now in much better condition than it was before its meal. And of course, it has an anus large enough for the insertion of a Pasteur pipette.

The weight of a female, whilst she is feeding, can become two hundred times greater. This eccentric dilation is possible as her abdomen lacks significant amounts of chitin.

The tick's stomach lining is made up of lateral sacs, which allow it to store oceanic quantities of blood. A complete meal is certainly a mission. It can take from three days to six weeks, which could become several years if the parasite penetrates more deeply in a natural cavity of its host.

Solitary, waiting in a tree, hidden in long grasses or tucked under the earth after a bush or a forest fire, which in turn hastens its hatching and increases its virulence, the tick, lacking eyes, ears, and voice, appears to be quite unprovided for. But its genetic code can do without these particulars and encourages it to feel body heat and to sniff the blood of animals or humans, from miles away, on which it may nourish itself.

. Industrious sorceress. It advances inexorably towards us, taking one step after another in the direction indicated by its interior compass, to provide us with its jackpot of disaster.

It attaches itself to the most accessible parts of its

target.

As it makes contact with the dampness of skin, its legs loose numbness and the mechanism of salivation is activated. It thrusts its sucking trunk in where the skin is most tender, preferably where it is warm and where there is shelter. The back of the ears, the skull covered with hair, the penis, the large lips of the vulva, groin and axilla are good anchoring points for ticks.

The saliva of the arthropod contains mostly vasodilators and anticoagulating agents as already mentioned, and a cocktail of immuno-suppressants (Richard Titus, Harvard School of Public Health).

Do chronic victims bitten by insects suffer from a gap in their cutaneous defence system, or present better receptors for the proteins contained in the saliva of the aggressor?

Why do certain human races not develop tick-bite fever?

Why is multiple sclerosis not usually found amongst the African racial groups?

Is this a matter of secular immunity?

These little pointed heads, shiny and black, transform themselves into leather-resembling pouches, capable of causing their hosts to lose a large quantity of blood if given the time. A single cow is at risk of losing up to 100 litres of blood per season. In the Kruger National Park for instance, 30 000 ticks were counted on a single buffalo.

In exchange for this meal, the tick, with or without a

business card, drops a few seeds of disease. The parasites will finally arrive at a satisfactory destination and will slowly but surely establish their domain in the body of the host, to the best of their ability.

Sharing the devastating activity of the tick, there are also fleas, lice, mites and other acaridae, which nourish themselves with the same discretion, reinforced in this instance by human dignity ignoring their presence.

On the list of these undesirable creatures there is also the small acarius, which transmits scabies.

The louse, once infected will remain so for its entire life. However, it does not transmit its entire infectious abundance to its offspring. The rickettsial agent is inherited, but not the spirochetes, which are only found in the eggs. The adult form will become infected at random during its promenades.

In ticks, trans-ovarian transmission of rickettsia can also be observed (Giroud et al).

The increased use of insecticides has decreased the amount of tick-eating and insect eating birds, which has increased the quantity of reservoirs containing rickettsiae and favoured its conservation. One way or another, with or without leitmotif, rickettsia is present.

In the next subdivision of this sort of morbid actuality, one rediscovers haemoglobin-sucking insects' fresh or dry ejections, which contain pathogens.

Tiresome flies and occasionally even mosquitoes are

also distributors.

Depending on the bias of the infected excrements, the cutaneous point of entry is extended to other equally effective, yet more concealed, obvious areas, such as the respiratory, digestive, and ocular tracts.

By infecting domestic pets or hunting trophies, rickettsia, chlamydia and mycoplasma are thus transmitted to man as well as to animals, and these in turn provide man with fresh meat and milk, thereby infecting him by passing through the digestive system.

As an example of infection via the ocular and respiratory passages, let us consider a goat ready to give birth in natural surroundings. This goat is a carrier of ticks and fleas, and will leave behind her one or more placentas, as do all herbivores. These placentas will soon be dried by the sun and reduced to dust by the wind. The dust produced has direct access to respiratory organs and the open eyes of a passer-by. If his mouth is open wide enough, there is direct access to the digestive system. During this expedition, any abrasions on the surface of the skin may form a cutaneous passage. And, added to that, if a dog accompanies him, it will surely find some afterbirth bits to swallow. After digestion, its freight of rickettsia will be renewed.

These guaranteed anonymous modes of transmission are valid for antelopes, rodents, bovines and all other quadrupeds, especially herbivores, that are often carriers of rickettsia or para-rickettsia.

This answers any queries, which may arise when, in

the absence of a tick or other bite, a patient presents with the disease as demonstrated by the following case histories of patients who have seen me for consultations.

This lawyer has no contact at all with nature. He has never seen a rat; the rodent itself has no intention either of meeting him, as it is more interested in his food. It leaves behind, on the kitchen table or on the Metro's door handles to be touched the following morning, fresh excretory products and faecal matter, which are not always visible, but virulent via cutaneous, ocular, respiratory or digestive pathways.

This jaded businessman is no longer able to get rid of his stress by playing golf, his favourite sport. Yet, the surrounding land is so enjoyable, with its river running along the northern side, and a hill acting as shelter from the dominant winds. The lawn could not be in better condition. It does not worry anyone that, because of its opulence, it was once used as a pasture to fatten up magnificent cattle, with their royal horns and imposing goitres. These animals constituted a treat for the myriads of ticks whose numerous germs infested the fresh droppings.

The odour dissipated, but not the contamination.

In addition to this, the perfect green of the golf course is maintained by spreading compost of animal origin and chemical fertilisers optimise this effect. The one gives a leg up to the other, to help conquer the immune system of anyone inhaling the apparently fresh air.

This professional young man knew that he was seriously ill.

After having consulted a specialist in internal medicine without success, he came to me and gave me a full description of his implacable fatigue. One morning, as he forced himself to pursue his career, apparently taken by a feeling of unease, he got out of his car and was run over by a big truck. I was unable to tell him about the results of his blood tests, which were strongly positive.

This camper is well aware of the danger ticks constitute; therefore, he maintains an impeccable hygiene every time he exposes himself.

Which is also the case when considering the example of a hiker. Both cover themselves meticulously with Baygon spray products, which are known for their efficiency. At night, with the aid of tweezers and disinfectants, they conscientiously detach the few shameless ticks, which may have taken shelter in the warm folds of the groin. So that the parasites will have no time to infect them with tick-bite fever.

Therefore they cannot understand why they are subject to a feeling of fatigue, which deepen progressively.

In the waiting room of my medical suite, I catch sight

of a massive burly man from behind. He is here to make his first appointment. I hear his warm voice telling the secretary that he is coming to please his wife. She has been complaining lately that he has become more difficult to live with and uncommonly depressed.

"In fact," he explains, "I have all the reasons to be depressed. My nights are too short and my days overloaded. I am a pastor and have four children to feed. In addition, I am suffering from insomnia..."

In this way he begins an interminable discourse, regularly interrupted by a hearty laugh and the sound of his hastily chewing biltong from a packet under his left arm.

"This is my drug," he says with a smile, "I can no longer do without it. The more I eat it, the more I need it. It is as if I have to immediately replace the energy I have just eaten."

Biltong or jerky is a kind of raw meat that has been dried and spiced before being consumed, as it is in South Africa. It is regarded as a luxury product. Caring mothers give it to their children to wean them off their milk and to assist in helping them to cut their first teeth.

This patient, who is a family member and friend, is continuing to heal. He fell sick during a holiday in Brazil. After following my treatment for one year, his state of health improved remarkably. Lately a strange

169

soreness has seized his hands again, which is a great nuisance as he is a sculptor. To maintain good physical and mental form, he devotes himself to horse riding in the forest near Brussels, and spends many hours grooming his horse and reinfecting himself.

This young woman started a commercial venture exporting zebra hides from South Africa to the USA. Despite her great fatigue and headaches, she continues to inspect them all, one by one. In this way, she has daily contact with skins still fresh with flea eggs and tick excrement.

Another patient becomes sick every time she unpacks statuettes made of animal hides and Raffia, coming straight from the Congo to her business. Clearly, the source of infection is inhalation.

The ecology Professor's occupation involves often scouring bush and veld. He suffers from peculiar pains that stab at his heart and render him incredibly tired. He is unable to concentrate, this brilliant Professor. The consulted specialists have only found a sedimentation rate that is slightly elevated and a barely perceptible leucopoenia. A diagnosis of mental depression has been suggested, with appropriate treatment.

His wife knows that his abundant night sweats have another origin. They came to consult me. After months, which lengthened into years of antibiotic treatment, he got back into shape. Due to his occupation, he will need subsequent treatment, as will his daughter, since he regularly brings ticks home from his trips. She has inherited his passion for the bush and the aptitude for being systematically bitten by infected ticks.

At each visit, "How many treatments do I still need?" he asks. "More or less?" he adds, to soften his imperative tone.

This defiance of logic is famous in my medical practice.

This man owns a crocodile farm, which makes demands on more energy than he has at the moment. He cannot imagine that the sound life he is leading in contact with these carriers of chlamydia is the basis of his weariness. He only lives with them, merely breeding them, treats their diseases professionally and performs bloody slaughter on them, at 35 °C and 100% humidity.

This young lady consults me, to please her mother whom I had treated with great success. She has had immense bouts of urticaria for a few months, which have resisted treatments prescribed by a number of different dermatologists consulted. There was nothing particular about her medical history, except the dermatological lesion which developed six months previously and was treated as eczema — without success.

The cutaneous biopsy, which followed, revealed the presence of scabies, a skin disease transmitted by small arachnids, which are equally carriers of rickettsia. In medical literature, this disease is associated with poverty and lack of hygiene.

This man, 50 years of age, consulted me because he had been told that I was an expert on recalcitrant pains. His right hip was torturing him night and day ever since he had undergone three hip replacements following bad falls.

"Why the falls?" I asked him.

"That has nothing to do with the reason for my visit," he answered evasively." I have fallen regularly for many years and more often recently ... I have been suffering from multiple sclerosis since I was 20. My sense of balance disappeared immediately following a tick bite, which gave me headaches for years.

The wife of a 50-year-old man cannot understand her husband's present condition. After being bitten by a dirty fat rat in London, he had suddenly lost his memory. The wound at his heel had cleared with the aid of antibiotics, but his children's names had disappeared from his mind. He could not remember to turn off taps and stub out cigarettes.

His blood tests showed very high levels of antibodies against three rickettsial antigens and two chlamydial antigens. Likewise, his auto-immune factors were increased and his white blood cell counts low. After a few months of treatment, he died of a heart attack, without being fortunate enough to have regained his memory. For those that knew him, he was an Alzheimer sufferer.

The origin of this disease remains complex.

This pianist never takes walks in the countryside and hates animals that, moreover, he finds dirty. His only passion is his piano, to which he devotes all his time. Since when has he been so depressed? Everything is going well in his world of successful concerts and diligent pupils. The only serious irritation that he cannot get rid of is the right piano pedal. It wedges itself too often due to the infiltration of dust.

"It is rat droppings," he says, as though he were sharing a secret.

A beautiful, clever and caring housewife has a hard time recognising the progressive changes happening to her three children. Her husband, a well-loved headmaster in a Johannesburg private school, will soon give up his job to try to understand and solve this incredible misfortune going on in his family.

Firstly, one of their two daughters, although excelling as much as her sister at school, brutally deteriorates in her performance.

"It is normal, all students go through highs and lows," a concerned teacher explains. "When one of two sisters finds herself on the crest of a wave, the other may very well be in a trough."

The young girl complains of headaches, and collapses on her bed on returning home from school. She talks less and less to her sister, unless to bicker.

"Often, teenage whims resemble diseases," says a logical and reassuring teacher.

" Maybe she's not given enough attention and feels a bit intimidated by her sister, who is always noisier and more exuberant than she is."

The first psychiatrist consulted confirms this fact. He does not realise the gravity of the situation. "But," he adds, "she will need medical treatment to get her out of this oncoming silence."

A few months go by. All involved wait patiently. There is no result. Except that her condition is worsening. The school has had enough of her.

She begins to formulate bizarre signals with her 10 fingers, which follow an invisible trajectory during the next hours. Her lips converse without an interpreter. If one attempts to reason with her, she locks herself in her room after throwing a tantrum. She is violent, she, who has a gentle nature.

The psychiatrist, to whom the panic-stricken parents have dragged her yet again, has let the word schizophrenia slip out. This echoes as a death sentence would, to the ears that have heard it.

The atmosphere in the house tenses up, the happiness is gone.

The sisters quarrel with each other and with their older brother.

Two years later, the second daughter also becomes impossible.

One understands how hard it must be to accept that one member of the family is demented. She is comforted. But nothing can make her hear reason. The school complains to the overwhelmed parents.

How should one deal with these tantrums, which are occurring more and more frequently?

She starts talking in an incoherent manner; she abandons the logical world. Back to the psychiatrist.

The same diagnosis is pronounced, the same treatment is given. The parents are forcefully interrogated concerning the mental state of other family members.

"They are not admitting to anything", thinks the psychiatrist, irritated.

But admit to what, as there are no abnormalities on the mother's side.

"So would it come from my husband's side?" the mother questions, slipping an oblique glance. But the husband also denies any abnormalities.

Behind his white coat, the psychiatrist has not changed his mind.

"Schizophrenia has often been considered as a genetic disease," insists the professional. "We are certainly in the presence of a confirmation of this hypothesis."

The brother can no longer handle the sound of his

parents discussing the matter too loudly; he can no longer stand seeing his sisters in this state. He is tired, depressed. He feels as though he must flee this misery, as quickly as possible, and everything will be well again.

He is offered a job in the town of Melbourne, Australia, where his cousins already are established. What an opportunity. He will take it, of course. Go and live on another continent. How lucky he is. If only he could feel less fatigued. Maybe it is due to the aspirin, which he is forced to take in large quantities, for his continual headaches.

What is the name of this disease causing headaches and madness, which has already been read about somewhere, already been published on too large a scale not to have had many readers?

Can the geneticist ignore the notion of environment to the extent of forgetting its existence?

This surgeon, on the other hand, deeply absorbed in his profession, declares, with confidence, that he has never seen rickettsia on the tip of his scalpel.

There, everything is in order and the ghost continues its crazy race, touching in its path several members of the same community or of the same family.

It strikes many of those who are involuntarily exposed. Most of them go on with their lives, handicapped in a more or less serious way. One meets them now and again, in search of the source of their embarrassment, in medical, nutritional or religious spheres. Several of them change their lifestyles entirely.

Anyway, the choice of healing is not always given to them. Therefore, sooner or later, they resign themselves to the fate that is encumbering them.

This disease is nothing but damnation. Some die or lose their sanity. Others, like myself, believing in the existence of the disease are castigated for it.

Now all that is needed is for those who are better equipped to undertake a large study of the environmental diseases.

Let us imagine that this research systematically uses the same biological screening for patients that present with similar symptoms, and that the results suggest that the symptoms have an infectious origin. Symptoms that have been thought to have a hereditary origin.

Or, how does one recognise the previous passage of an infectious agent in today's diseases?

Logically, this information will be followed by treatment, a treatment that is efficient and reproducible on a scale as ample as the distribution of the disease.

All these apparently imaginary, chronic and incurably sick people, would then no longer depend on their medical insurances or on their surroundings, or be miserable recipients of public assistance, but would form part of the productive and content people of our society. This is a simple economic suggestion.

One would need to reformulate insurance questionnaires.

Granted, they all contain questions on the previous family medical history of each applicant. This is done to limit the accessibility of insurance cover for clients who may have had an ancestor who was the victim of diseases such as multiple sclerosis, myocardial infarction, Parkinson's, nervous depression, rheumatoid and other auto-immune infections. Are these, in fact, more hereditary than malaria?

Does one not find the same collection of hereditary and infectious conditions necessary for the infection to develop in the midst of the same family? The contact with the intermediates — fleas lice and ticks — is equally likely for each member of the household.

Should insurance cover be declined or loaded for environmental diseases?

"Here, Mr Dupont, your serology is positive for two types of rickettsia, one mycoplasma, two chlamydia and bilharzia. Your white cells count is elevated and the same for your sedimentation rate. Your iron level is about non-existent. Were you unaware of these results?"

"Absolutely. How is that possible? My doctor frequently performs thorough blood investigations. He even checks my cholesterol level every six months."

(This conversation was disclosed from confidential files with Mr Dupont's permission.)

For the few thousand patients who have consulted me up until now, reporting all kinds of symptoms of which fatigue is always one, this diagnostic approach concerning intracellular micro-organisms forms part of my routine. It gives me information that, to me, is much more valuable in relation to their health, present and future, than a cholesterol test.

More and more often I come across cases where rickettsial, chlamydia and mycoplasma infections affect the whole family. If at first sight, it seems strange that an entire family is ill simultaneously, this is in fact more logical than it is extraordinary.

A few years ago, a patient consulted me for hepatic dysfunction that had been present for the two preceding years. A hepatic biopsy only revealed fatty infiltration, without specifying its origin.

My diagnosis, based on symptomatology and blood tests, was one of a rickettsial disease, accompanied by mycoplasma, chlamydia and bilharzia.

Some days later his wife consulted me, complaining of great fatigue. The next day she brought me her two children, aged six and eight, as she found them to also be tired.

Was I in the presence of a hypochondriacal mother hen? No, at that time I simply lacked family medical experience.

The whole family appeared to be sporty, young and in good health. And all four had the same infectious serology, which was positive, accompanied by hepatic dysfunction, iron deficiency and slight leucopoenia.

After three months of antibiotic treatment administered in a pulsated and alternating fashion, the two children recovered. This was confirmed by a blood test, which showed normal hepatic functioning. The serum had satisfactory iron levels, without having prescribed supplements, and the white blood cells were restored.

The same thing happened for the mother six months later.

As for the father, after verifying that his general condition had improved, as had his hepatic function, I could only advise him to continue the treatment as he and his family were emigrating to Australia.

I recall another example, one of a patient who was about 40 years old and had been suffering from multiple sclerosis, intense fatigue, dreadful migraines and cardiac dysfunction for 10 years. Not by coincidence, her blood tests were positive regarding rickettsia, chlamydia and mycoplasma. I hold these three responsible for the disappearance of her iron stores and the rise in the count of her thyroid antibodies, as well as her rheumatoid factor.

Her eldest daughter was 15; she was suffering similarly from abnormal fatigue, loss of balance, Raynaud's syndrome, scotomas, and from shortness of breath. These forced her to stop participating in school sporting competitions. I was able to establish that her blood test results were identical to her mother's.

The second daughter was 12. She had the same list of clinical disorders, in all aspects as her sister, with the same blood test results.

Finally there was the youngest, a son of 10 years, who had superb blue eyes. Surely not sick, this one too? In response to this, obviously there has to be a logical explanation: if he has come to see me, it is not for the pleasure of meeting me, nor to travel a 1 000 kilometres in a sweltering car sweating beneath the iron roof that absorbs the sun's heat, nor for want of spending the little money that his parents' farm makes, nor because he wishes to see a fat needle being planted into his arm.

So what is he complaining of? That he has fainted on many occasions, that he was hospitalised thereafter, that his trouble was investigated without success. His head aches and his heart throbs so forcefully in his chest that he is incapable of running. The time has come for you to cover me in ridicule as I put it in black and white: He tested positive for rickettsia, chlamydia and mycoplasma.

All at once, I feel faint. I would like to escape, forget everything and return to the operating theatre where everything is calm and efficient. There, where nobody complains. There, where one is not harassed nor jeered at. There where slanderers believe in burying what must be buried, before building the walls of a court case around one…

But let's return to our little patient. During the auscultation, he presented an impressive heart murmur that no one had told him about. I advised the mother to get a cardiologist's opinion, or to have an ultrasound taken to see the state of his cardiac valves.

In the meantime, after five sets of antibiotic treatment, the heart murmur disappeared and the patient appeared to be full of life. The appointment with the cardiologist, who was a very busy man and had been unable to accommodate the patient for a further two weeks, was cancelled.

Perhaps you would like to know what happened to the two sisters. The younger one is in good health, thank you doctor. And the elder one, although her test results are improving, is still in need of my care.

I have but a brief comment concerning the mother's state of being: her condition, including her test results, is slowly improving after six months of treatment. Her sense of balance is recovering and she suffers less frequently from headaches. I have not seen her for three months. Last week, she phoned me to explain her absence: her mother was dying of cancer, there was work to be done on the farm and the family was in financial difficulty. Nevertheless, she feels much better.

The pathological agent that seizes all my unfortunate patients is endowed with extraordinary virulence. It is resistant to humidity as well as to drought. It maintains its infectious powers for as long as 60 days in milk, for up to four months in sand, up to six months in meat and up to nine months in cotton. (Published by S. Nicolau and A. Mas Barnard in 1963, in the Bulletin de la Société de Pathologie Exotique.)

From Europe to Africa, from America to Australia and going down to New Zealand and passing through Asia, vectors are present. They are propagated through the continents, thereby hybridising due to the migrating birds that have always been host to insects.

Homer, in the sixth section of the Iliad, speaks of the "migration of gulls, who every winter carry the carnage and war from one end of the earth to the other".

Recently the great increase in air traffic and the modernising of transport has assured the vectors of global geographic enterprise, in those countries where their activities are not knocked out by the Antarctic cold.

I had almost forgotten to mention fish, which also share the burden of harbouring these detestable commensals (Paul Giroud). There one must be wary of those delicious dishes that come from traditional Japanese cuisine, in case they are made from raw fish.

Even though my reputation is at stake, I have to extend my list of rickettsia carriers to oysters. Found in the rocky depths, they function as marine filters. Thus they retain in their fleshy bodies the numerous impurities that dawdle in the ocean. After this, we eat them.

And now, all that is really left for me to do is to blame the grey dust clouds of a variety of origins that empty out their emanations as they sprinkle over our wheat fields.

CHAPTER 9:

PATHOGENICITY

*"What we claim to be an accident is and
can only be the ignored consequence
of a known effect."*
—Philosophical dictionary—

Readers do not stop here.

The play carries on.

There is more chance it will become a two-partner
fight in so far as the stage actors are still able to take
part. It will depend on a legion of changing circumstances and a few predictable factors. Among them, the
quality of food dispensed by the host to the parasite,
just like the food a child picks up from his plate will
determine his smile and his growth; and a minimum of
consideration from the parasite for the vital function of
its sponsor without whom everything has to start

again.

What a painful feeling of suspense: which is going to destroy the other?

Is it necessary to resort to murder? Which method to use? A surprise attack, a dazzling strike, or a cold war-type of battle, smouldering in the system for long and painful years.

The strike is the acute phase. It comes like a disaster, or may even pass unnoticed.

Then comes the slow phase. It settles much more quickly in our system than physiological old age. Even then, mistakes are common.

After penetrating the host it was lucky enough to find, the micro-organism will come to blows and survive a chain of unexpected incidents, which could cost it its life at any moment.

Because of its poor biological equipment, it cannot find all its nutrients in the blood stream.

It must act swiftly. Since the current is strong even when the blood pressure is low.

All other kinds of mechanisms oppose its presence: temperature starts to rise and becomes unbearable, white cells jump from everywhere, antibodies bomb its antigens, and other allies less specific but just as dangerous, deploy such as antinuclear factors, C reactive proteins, kinases...

So much energy released to revert to square one.

Carried along in the blood stream, it will be surrounded by vascular cells as soon as it arrives in the human body. The first lining of these vessels is called endothelium.

Maybe this initial contact will cause it to cross the cell membrane. The rubbing process stimulates the production of some enzymes which will help its mooring and this would explain its affinity for endothelial cells.

In a bid to survive, it attends to the most powerful urge. After adhesion to the cell membranes, it penetrates the endothelium after being engulfed by cellular extensions.

This phenomenon, known as phagocytosis, will guide the germ straight into the cytoplasm itself.

Well done.

Again, there it is, sound and healthy. Even if it is only a temporary rest.

Numerous publications describe this affinity of rickettsiae for the endothelial system. Currently, the vascular endothelium is no longer considered to be a lining of cells only, but because of the production of nitric acid and other vasoactive substances, it is recognised as an essential organ of our bodies.

Impairment of its function, because of invasion by microorganisms, will undoubtedly play a major role in human pathology.

The bugs' colonising activities in the cytoplasm of the endothelial cell are no different to those seen elsewhere in nature. This means simply eating and multiplying. To achieve this, they toss down electrolytes, glucose, proteins and minerals from the host.

Easy to imagine the damage created in the cell by the rickettsial bud. To survive, the germs use the cell's metabolic pathways, bypass and paralyse the energy supply from the blood to the different organs.

And so easy to prove. For example, by testing the concentration of magnesium, sugar, iron, and globulins in the blood.

On top of this hijacking of raw material, they commit the offence of occupying the endothelial cell itself. Therefore, they prevent this organ from playing its key role, namely regulation of physiological exchanges between the blood stream and the rest of the body.

How can the free flow of electrolytes, minerals, and oxygen happen from the blood stream to the endothelial cell in one direction, and of carbohydrates and other toxins from the working tissues (muscle, brain, or other) via the endothelial cell in the other direction? How chaotic! And now, in the middle of this stampede, who said that the traffic lights of the alarmed body would be functioning?

How heavy is the fatigue emanating from cells suffocating after lack of oxygen. This is almost as if someone stood on the oxygen pipe of a patient in ICU, producing a partial obstruction and an indecisive death.

Paul Giroud described rickettsiae as real vascular

sponges, paralysing everything; leechlike little by little, the vessel disintegrates, the brain becomes soaked with toxins, muscle melts, myelin disappears, the bone's surface looses its polish and necrotic tissue accumulates.

Now comes the time for reproduction, by binary fission inside the cytoplasm of endothelial cells, as we have already mentioned.

This creates a distension of the cell membrane to bursting point. The cell is torn, and the rickettsial corpuscles are flung into the blood stream.

The host's alarm devices are again activated: they are called inflammatory mechanisms. Fever rages and comes down, patients perspire profusely, headaches flare up, hearts race and joints swell.

Again, some blood tests as well as some instruments such a thermometer, a stethoscope or just the human eye will pick up the reactions.

In the bloodstream, rickettsiae will present as undeveloped forms and mature forms. Undeveloped forms do not have the ability to penetrate the cell, nor to survive in the blood flow. Therefore, they disappear.

Mature forms again use their ability to be phagocytosed by the macrophage. It brings about new colonies of free rickettsiae in the cytoplasm and the round is perpetuated.

Sometimes, luckily or not, a parasite will be found in a vacuole, a kind of bubble produced in the cytoplasm. Leashed in that way, its growth and its multiplication are slowed down, and in a living nightmare, this horrid creature will take on the behaviour of the Sleeping Beauty of our childhood. Never mind the lack of beauty, the much more important difference is that its sleep will not last for 100 years.

What produces this vacuole? The germ or the host?

The biological changes produced by their migration from a vessel's lumen through tissue, using blood as a vehicle, is no different to that seen during a conflict, when enemies invade our land.

It is a state of war, famine, pain, hypoglycaemias of all kind, and the resistance network tightens up.

Pathologists witness a tremor in the macrophage T population, called natural killers. But rickettsiae are known to paralyse macrophages at the site of action. This will reduce the hosts' defence mechanism.

Besides that, production of cytokines will start; not only do they have antigenic properties, but they also produce vasoconstriction, allergies and the dismantling of the nerve myelin, as Paul Legag described a few decades ago.

It is a supernatural role.

Their effects are often taken as the cause of the symptoms.

Not all that rush of cytokines happens without creating strange body aches, amazing allergies, or weird neurological symptoms.

Because science is beautified when precise, I will mention the circulation of three types of cytokines:

endotoxins that can cause pain, allergens that can trigger allergies, and neurotoxins producing neurological imbalance.

The immune system, exhausted by this overproduction of antibodies, becomes short of breath.

Sometimes, its devastated storerooms generate incendiary shortcuts.

The immune system's production of antibodies carries on, without recognition of the bugs as stimulus. The confused host attacks itself by producing elevated levels of so-called rheumatoid and antinuclear factors, as well as elevated levels of C reactive protein and thyroid antibodies. The thyroid, the joints, the intestine, the neurological tissues are caught in the cross fire, bombarded by antibodies, and go through a self-destructive process. The patient steps into the classification of auto-immune disease.

All along the rickettsial trajectory, sheets like peritoneum, the pleura, the pericardium, the epiploic membrane and the vagina mucosae become inflamed and start exudation.

What vitriol for the system.

This engulfing of the vascular territory will not pass unnoticed. A general vasculitis may take place, reversible or not.

Realising that we are a vascular system from top to toe, our infectious affair is far from over.

It is time to move on to the next chapter.

CHAPTER 10:

EVOLUTION OF RICKETTSIAL DISEASES

"Whatever nature brings about,
It will not appear brusquely."
—*Gustave Flaubert*—

To go from cellular invasion to the assault of the entire human system, micro-organisms need more time than one would imagine.

Luck is also compulsory.

How many generations were sacrificed for the survival of this little festival of disturbances? Twisted up in bundles of blood vessels, leading to the death of some and the reincarnation of others.

All waves are not favourable.

But once introduced into the cellular structure of the

body, this parasite, which has an affinity for the vascular system, falls into a gold mine. Namely: the omnipresence of this system in our body. Every one of our organs depends on it. The possibility of invasion of our territory by these microscopic organisms has no other restriction.

What a multitude of ports of arrival. The cerebral artery and all its connections, the ponto-cerebral, the optic chiasma and its palpebral, nasal and frontal branches, the deep lingual and its tortuous path, the tympanic membrane with its buzzing corridors, the anonymous artery bowing before the trachea, the diploïc, the red aortic arch swinging brand new oxygen that rises then curves dorsally and then lands at the navel, the carotid and its follies, the jugular, the two coronaries, one sinistra and the other dextra, the vena cava always represented in blue, the thoracic and the abdominal vein, the circumflex vein hidden behind the appendix found on the left of the enigmatically named auricle , the lumbar, the azygos and then the portal vein.

This is but a rough draft of the vascular labyrinth of the human species.

To know more, one should procure the Grant's Atlas of Anatomy and follow rickettsiae's head start under an anatomo-pathological light.

Apparently, there are no important frontiers to cross.

It suffices to allow itself to be carried by the blood whirlpool, either freely or in the form of a small embolism accidentally detached from the vascular lining. If from time to time a resistance that is too well orchestrated looms, the formula parasites-in-association will come to the end of it.

The paradise of the ones pushes the others in hell.

Consequently, according to the assaulted vessel, or other vessels, the symptoms will vary in unusual constellations. This is what is baffling about the chronically fatigued.

Along the course of invasion, one group of blood vessels might be more seriously damaged than others. The tissue that is nourished by these blood vessels may develop signs of disease that will be given a name that is more conventional medically than the name CFS.

Here is a proposal of the list:
- In the first place, CFS and its Siamese twin, fibromyalgia, two diseases that are caused directly by the cellular anoxia due to the presence of parasites inside of the cell.

- Cardio-vascular diseases, of which the onset may be abrupt or insidious.
From time to time, a valve may need to be replaced or a by-pass may be executed. Thus, in a headlong flight, which could have been avoided, an atheromatous plaque is urgently removed, as it is about to provoke a myocardial infarction, which is also wrongly called a heart 'attack'. Rickettsiae do not strike hearts,

as termites do not blast trees.

Our micro-organisms have similarly been described as causing myocarditis, endocarditis, pericarditis as well as vascular aneurisms (Paul Giroud).

A pilot study recently conducted in Italy bears witness to the reduction of coronary relapses in patients treated with antibiotherapy after myocardial infarcts.

Certain types of hypertension probably originate from the same pathological source. In fact, a number of our patients suffering from hypertension and fatigue, who have been treated with antibiotherapy, over a few years, saw their blood pressure normalise after a short period of treatment.

In vascular blows, one must quote Raynaud's syndrome, involving the small sized arteries and resembling a chill of the tissues, and Buerger's disease, leading to the partial or complete obstruction of a blood vessel, which ultimately leads to death. The inflammatory escort of arterial, venous and nervous suffering is present in these two conditions.

● Neurological diseases caused by rickettsia and chlamydia are the subject of copious publications. Among these are multiple sclerosis, epilepsy, Parkinson's disease, Guillain Barré and attention deficit disorder or hyperactive children. These germs have been isolated from the cerebro-spinal fluid of patients suffering from multiple sclerosis.

● Various psychotic disorders and a number of psychiatric diseases, ranging from imperceptible depression to violent schizophrenia, are explained by 'chronic vascular rickettsial encephalitis.' (Philippe Bottero)

● Pulmonary disorders, which start as pneumonia or pleurisy and perpetuate as an unforgivable barking cough without forgiveness for the circadian cycle, can be attributed to rickettsial diseases and more classically to chlamydia pneumoniae.

● Diseases of the digestive system, such as appendicitis, pseudo appendicitis, due to mesenteric adenopathy, coeliac disorders, Crohn's disease, etc, could find the same origin, although in humans the link with intracellular infections and digestive disorders has not been studied as precisely as that with cardiac and nervous disorders.

Veterinary science has noted it.

Yet it would be easy to do so in medicine. Organs removed daily from anaesthetised bodies form the material theoretically dreamed of for similar studies.

I can only recall one such publication: the presence of chlamydias in children suffering from acute appendicitis. This condition presented as an epidemic in a school situated along Lake Kivu in Rwanda. Paul

Giroud reported this incident in 1979, in the Bulletin de l'Academie Nationale de Médecine.

To illustrate the possibility of a progressive rickettsial impact, I have often been struck by the medical life of a worldwide celebrity. Twenty years ago this man was an amateur alpine climber and canoeist. He was without a doubt in good health. In the early 90s, an article in a South African magazine announced that he was suffering from a strange disease, which included great fatigue and muscular pains. His movements were painful. The disorder in question was a rare bacterial one. It resembled CFS so much that I could not stop myself from phoning one of his contact numbers in Pretoria. It's not difficult to understand that no attention whatsoever was given to me. I was not counting on it anyway. I did it only for peace of mind. A Paris Match in 1998 displayed a series of photos of this famous man resting in the mountains for the sixth consecutive year, said the commentary, during the month of July. His white clothes floated lazily in the grass and brought out the vegetation's rich and provocative green colour.

Rich in what?

Already present was the tremble in his left hand: Parkinson's disease.

Some time later, an article reported that at the age of 76, our hero was going to undergo surgical intervention, fortunately nothing serious: appendicitis.

More recently, before a crowd of youths gathered from across the world to applaud him, he could not repress his trembling and his exhaustion.

● Amongst ocular diseases of rickettsial origin we find uveites, retinal angiopathies and ophthalmic neuritis. Trachoma of chlamydial origin plunges a large part of humanity into permanent obscurity every day.

● At the level of the liver, these micro-organisms cause a singular toxicity leading to an enzymatic elevation and fatty infiltration.

● At the level of the spleen, they can cause splenomegaly, a swelling of the organ, which will often become the object of surgical ablation.

● Renal infections have been described.

● At a gynaecological level, one finds successive abortions, endometriosis, and coagulation disorders, with an elevated level of cardiolipin antibodies.

● On a prostate level, infections are frequent.

● The testis can become inflamed and swell in a similar way to that of guinea pigs inoculated with typhus. (See added photo)

● Cutaneous lesions, petechial or haemorrhagic, are found in most rickettsial cases. They are accompanied by extreme fatigue, headaches and perspirations.

We are lucky enough to witness the disappearance of the numerous cutaneous lesions with antibiotherapy.

It can take only a few months for ulcers found on legs, present for a number of years, to disappear.

Blemishes caused by hyper-pigmentation generally spread on the inside of the leg are erased; this is more frequently found in male patients.

Rashes of the butterfly type found on the face in cases of lupus, eczema and extended psoriasis can be easily suppressed with antibiotherapy.

One day a patient consulted me presenting with a rare case of Morphea's disease. This lady was in her forties and had been suffering from arthritic pains since adolescence. After school was time for a siesta, which sometimes lasted into the night. From time to time she would be awakened by violent headaches. Her mother was continually buying aspirin. At the age of 20, she had developed ulcerations on her arms and thighs. The ulcerations, instead of healing with medical treatment, sank to the muscular level. Her left leg was raw.

Antibiotics did not stem the infection. Doctors lost their patience and advised her to have the limb amputated. She needed a last opinion. My routine biological demands revealed a classic list composed of a variety of infectious diseases, accompanied by auto-immune factors that were on the whole positive, abnormal hepatic enzymes as well as an iron deficiency. Hoping to slow down the devouring harm, I administered my antibiotic treatment. A year later, the ulcers had taken on the aspect of whitish slabs, the blood analysis had normalised, the rheumatic pains were becoming more infrequent and her fatigue had disappeared. Logic can be astonishing sometimes.

Why was this disease named after the God of sleep?

Just as eccentric is the tale of a patient covered from head to toe in ulcers. The condition had started a few years before, following insect bites. So far, she has undergone five courses of seven days antibiotic treatments. Her ulcers are slowly disappearing.

How could the search for infectious disease become part of the routine investigation of each of these conditions? A search including as many strains of infectious and environmental agents as would-be. A screening that picks up different origins amongst the same disease. MS, arteriopathies, uveitis, rheumatologic diseases, miscarriages are obviously far from being all due to infection.

Now, the disease spreads: from being localised in organs to invading the entire system.

Causal agents have opened the doors. Henceforth they may rest and flounder in their second form, that is persistent latency. In this stage a few toxins are released from time to time. This explains the clinical setbacks, also called relapses, of systemic diseases.

According to our clinical experiences, some auto-immune diseases, such as rheumatoid and psoriasis arthritis, lupus, scleroderma, Sjögren's disease, etc, are often due to rickettsiae and associated germs.

Then again, most patients suffering from MS present with auto-immune biological ailments. For example, amongst my patients, Hashimoto disease is commonly seen in association with multiple sclerosis. Is this pure coincidence? Why should neurologists look for thyroid antibodies?

However, some patients present simultaneously with many diseases. Or one after another.

The following associations are regular: rheumatoid arthritis and depression; ocular and gynaecological diseases; lupus and heart attacks; appendicitis and high blood pressure, liver disorder and MS.

Alternatively, one patient suffering from ME may develop MS, and another patient presenting with a case of MS may have a greater chance of dying of a heart attack, if left untreated.

It seems to be nothing but different stages of the same disease.

From the start, the person in question feels ill. A reaction is needed to reverse the situation. The lifestyle could be changed. Restoratives could be taken.

To lighten his exhaustion, the person may gulp down all sorts of vitamins and trace elements.

In the assailed flesh of our body, an increase in anabolic material concentrated in the blood will facilitate the germs' growth. This will constitute a direct aid to their prosperity.

For the pains and pathological inflammation, the patient will have painkillers, anti-inflammatories, cortisone and chemotherapy administered.

Thanks especially to the last two treatments, the patient's immune system will lose its remaining competency and the growth of the pathological agents will be even further enhanced.

As time passes, this patient, who is now genuinely sick, steers himself alternatively to a cardiologist, a rheumatologist, a neurologist, a surgeon, a gastroenterologist, a psychiatrist or an ophthalmologist, all depending on the dominating localisation of his aches.

Homeopaths, acupuncturists or iridologists may also form part of this pilgrimage.

The chosen practitioner will baptise the disease according to the turn it has taken. He will thus indefinitely close the door on the possibility of an infectious origin.

From now on the ailment is an entity made up of symptoms that are rightly its own. In tribute to these symptoms, the disease is classified and believed to be treatable.

These disturbing symptoms are taken as the aggressors. They will be eliminated. In fact fevers, pains, fatigue and palpitations are considered to be an attack on the body, rather than the body's defence mechanism against diseases.

For example fever, when it represents a corporal reaction against an invasion of germs, will drastically diminish the aggressors' longevity. This has been proven repeatedly, notably during the studies done in vitro on Schistosoma mansoni, which were published in 1963 in the Bulletin de la Société de Pathologie Exotique.

The symptoms are a manifestation of the disease, but they are not the disease. Conversely, symptoms are forcibly subjective. Medicine based on them cannot in itself be scientific. It is medicine driven by sensations.

Dwelling on the dominating sensations of the patient, he will be labelled with a certain syndrome. In turn the symptom will carry its schemer's name. Filed business: this patient is suffering from Creutzfeldt-Jakob, his neighbour shows Crest's syndrome, this one suffers from Crocodile's tears syndrome, that one from Carpal tunnel's syndrome, and another is struck by Charles Bonnet's syndrome. From Catatonia we move onto a Chinese restaurant as we pass by the Cri-du-chat.

Just as the fountain where Narcissus drowned himself, disheartened by his unattainable image, was not aware of his beauty.

"Was he (Narcissus) handsome?" the water asked the

flowers, who were mourning his death.

"But how could you not have noticed his appearance?" the flowers answered between sobs, "he was always near you."

"And yet I never looked at him," said the water, aghast. "Every time he paid me a visit, I was searching for my own reflection in his eyes."

In the same light, that is where classification in medicine will lead us.

Medicine presumes it to be a conclusion and paralyses all access that an etiological approach could provide.

Let's get back to our symbiotic phantoms. These are transmitted either by a little tick innocently digesting our red blood cells, or by a louse stuffing itself with blood that bestows upon it wonderful fecundity.

Where are they headed in the masked ball of our violated body?

This is written in the stars.

It depends on them as well as on us.

Their virulence is not accidental, but the result of incessant mutations that have effectively triumphed over our defence systems through the centuries.

What is the state of the premises?

Our metabolism is genetically coded and will make us more or less favourable growth medias.

The presence of other parasites, shipping and

strengthening one another, the temperature, the light intensity, sound, electric waves, adrenaline discharges, chemical aggressions and the mysterious alchemy are but a few interacting factors in the course of the germs' evolution.

The germ's virulence can unbalance the bone marrow's composition and lead to all sorts of disorders. Pancytopoenias, anaemias, thrombocytopoenias, leucopoenias or even leukaemias have been described.

The bone marrow is struck by the brutality of the blows.

The same situation can be met by an assault that has lasted too long.

The infectious origin of this type of leukaemia does not stand much of a chance of being considered.

It's not an academic and sterile exercise to look for the why of things in medicine, because they are the key to the exit door.

No, do not put words in my mouth. Obviously leukaemia cannot be treated with tetracycline, even if there may be cases where it helps. I have seen patients being treated for atypical leukaemia, sometimes for a number of years, heal during the course of antibiotic therapy.

"Do anything, Doctor. Anyway, I have only three months to live," a despairing patient told me during his first visit. In his fifties, he sported a military uniform laden with stripes. He was suffering from broad discomfort, accompanied by a recalcitrant leucopoenia.

He was straining under the chemotherapy treatment.

A few months later, a booming voice challenged me over the phone.

"What have you done to General X? I do not see the point of your demand for biological tests. And where did you learn to treat leukaemia with antibiotics?"

"I treated him for a rickettsial infection," I replied to the specialist. As I was about to launch into a more detailed explanation, he interrupted me, becoming brusquely unnerved: "I really don't see any possible connexion between an infection and the leukaemia that the General is suffering from. He has been following your treatment for over six months. I was not aware of it. But anyway," he added, "it's without importance, as the white blood cell count has finally spontaneously normalised itself and he will not be consulting you anymore."

Then, probably happy to have said what he had to say, he softened and continued: "But to what end do you use so many antibiotics? Apparently you put all your patients on doses irreversibly toxic to the liver. Why?"

I'd been reduced to a youngster caught in a trap.

"That is how I treat them after having diagnosed them as suffering from rickettsial diseases." I replied patiently.

"Suffering from what?" he roared into the receiver, as if the anger that seized him was accompanied by a sudden deafness.

"From rickettsial infections," I resumed, with a perseverance that had been impressed on me by this type of question over the years.

"But," he yelled indignantly, "there is no rickettsia in this country!"

"Oh," I said, ready to hang up, "and what makes you say that?"

" It is simple," he retorted, " there's no test for it in South Africa."

I was about to give reasons for the veracity of this deficiency, but he deprived me of the opportunity.

A multiple infection of germs can lead by the same mechanism to paralysis of bone marrow function. In fact, one can very well imagine the reduction and disappearance of white blood cells under the weight of the numerous assailants.

The microorganism's chronic nature enables it to establish its long existence in the host cell.

This will set off changes at the level of the cell membrane's surface, where the micro-organisms are carpeted.

These changes could cause the sudden manifestation of two different mechanisms:

● The first would be the cell's changed surface being rejected by the body, which reacts against a seemingly foreign substance. In this case, the infection has taken the auto-immune disease's path and we find regularly a normalisation of auto-immune factors following adequate antibiotic therapy.

● In other cases, the host can accept the infected cells that have a different aspect now, with their changed surface membrane. The host may then produce a specific protein that allows him to swing the infected cells in his own genetic patrimony. Just as the original cells. This may have a direct consequence at the stage of mitosis: the production of cells having altered surface membranes. We are now in the presence of cloned cells that are disassembled, new and maybe anarchical.

Does that not correspond to the definition of a cancer?

In other words, it is possible that certain cancers are the result of an infectious disease. These cancers are therefore not an entry into the world of diseases, but the sequel to a pre-existing pathological disaster, that has changed or by-passed our defence systems.

Besides, this has already been written.

And there we are at the surgeon that, with his scalpel, is trying to repair the disaster. After him, it is to the oncologist, specialist in chemotherapy, that we pay a visit.

As this treatment takes effect, our patient enters a state of immune-suppression of the entire system. To eliminate the growth of cancerous cells, the growth of all cells is inhibited, including those involved in defence.

This situation seems dangerous for other infectious domiciles matted in the body in a dormant state. It is not untimely to suggest that this lack in defence could permit the reactivation of their virulence.

So what name would we classically give to this situation in the evolution of a cancer? Secondaries?

This has no other pretension than a timid suggestion. If I am arrogant enough to write it down, it's in the hope that this idea will be followed by a systematic anatomopathological study.

The end of this chapter is not intended to be a scientific assertion, but proposes to the reader a different approach where one forgets the name of a disease, and its symptomatic and other rigid criterias, in favour of the causative agent.

The smooth surface of the water inviting the peacock to flaunt is nothing but the false reflection of the distracted observer, to better conceal the instinct pushing him to strut. Similarly, the shadow cast by biochemical changes caused by germs, is but the umbrella under which the germs are sheltering, so that practitioners looking for the cause of the disease do not find the real culprit.

One could sometimes compare certain scientific research to a stroll in the star-shaped body of an octopus. Instead of staying in the centre of the animal, as it is there, logically, that everything is happening, the sightseer strays into one of the eight limbs. On arriving at the end of a limb, he strikes a dead end and has no choice but to double back. The centre of the octopus is the parasite and the limbs are only its extensions. It is often a waste of time to walk in the suburbs if you mean business in town.

It is when we have come face to face with evidence that we are led to the core of the investigation. But man has the troublesome habit of overlooking evidence. What hits him between the eyes seems to be too simple to represent reality.

CHAPTER 11:

THE DIAGNOSIS

"To play, one needs rules."
—*Y Delmas-Redigoutsos*—

Life has to be comfortable.

The diagnosis that I lay down for my patients must be too, as much as possible.

In order to establish it this way, I was lucky enough to have been given a few private lessons by all of my patients since 1992.

Today, I have reached a conclusion. Before being in a strategic position to convey a diagnosis, one must uphold the following four points, which are four forti-fied and complementary zones making up a polygon:

- The history of the disease
- The symptoms

- The clinical examination
- The biological tests

If one of these is missing, the polygon loses its familiar extremities, and the mechanism of approach becomes chaotic. Similar to a windswept carriage losing baggage as it rattles down the road, how can one formulate a diagnosis without taking all the data into consideration? This would be like entrusting the interpretation of the evidence to luck.

It has happened that doctors have asked my opinion on the results of their own patients' Micro-agglutination tests in order to arrive at a diagnosis.

About the test.

Stripped of its context. A technician without tools. Polychromes in black and white lay bare of all other pixels.

Unachievable.

In fact, this test is only one step in the mechanism set up to perceive the interacting elements. Without further information, its significance is limited, as is any biological result.

On its own, it is insufficient to expose all the secrets of a pathological rubble site.

Let's take, for example, a farmer in daily contact and intimacy with his animals. He feeds them, cares for them, slaughters them, touches them, inhales near them and eats them.

Every morning, as a healthy start, he fills his cereal bowl to the brim with fresh milk in readiness for the day's labours.

He is a great eater of fresh meat and is passionate about biltong — dried meat, which is left uncooked.

Suppose he has a brother who lives in town. His ultramodern and ultra clean apartment is situated on the sixth floor of a building, near his office where he practices law. Absorbed in his career, beset with problems to be solved, he has no contact with nature. Rats, indispensable pests, have not yet paid him a visit. He drinks only long-life milk, which doesn't expire for a minimum of two years, and biltong doesn't enter into his working schedule. He does not encumber himself with domestic pets.

Let's imagine that each brother has fathered a young child. The two brothers are healthy, as are their children.

Given the picture above, let's analyse each in the light of our four parameters:

- The 'history of the disease' compartment will be empty.
- They will not present any pathological symptoms.
- The clinical examination will probably be insignificant.
- Clinical biology will be within normal parameters.

Nothing is gained if one does not use Giroud's Micro-agglutination test in order to satisfy scientific curiosity. For the results' analyses to be complete, academically one could also bleed the two children.

Normally, different results would be achieved.

This is due to the fact that the farmer's immune system is incessantly being stimulated, while his brother's is not, or possibly is, but only occasionally.

The farmer's child has been in close and constant contact with antigens of rickettsial origin. On the contrary, his cousin will have encountered only a few, and later on in his life.

The antibodies' levels will demonstrate these differences.

In this specific case, if the farmer's serum did not contain antibodies, I would suspect that he did not respond to the stimulation of antigens to which he is exposed on a daily basis. He would thus present a state of immune decay.

Conversely, his brother's serum should signal weak positivity, an immune signature. It will be stable and little elevated against rickettsiae.

The farmer's child has all the right conditions for rapidly developing, strongly positive serology. Hopefully, this will not accompany the onset of illness.

The urban child's results should not be positive, unless he is still an infant and his mother has antibodies to transmit during the peri-natal period.

Here are four different results for four different people, all four in perfect health. Those results emanate from a precise science called Clinical Biology.

The final equilibrium is obtained only after adding agreements and substracting discordances.

Taking this fact into consideration, one cannot

comment on the positivity of Giroud's Micro-agglutination test, or interpret it as a pathological certainty if
isolated from its context. Lost in space and time, it is
only a sign of a previous exposure to rickettsiae. An
undoubted sign. It is left to the clinician to conduct an
inquiry based on this reliable foundation.

Here is another example of emanation, in which
plain serology can lead us: the test for bilharzia.

This disease is quite common in Africa and is due to
the presence of a parasitic fluke found in man's
muscular and circulatory system. Its systematic investigation forms part of my patients' records. Those who
present with suggestive symptoms and whose biological tests turn out positive are treated.

Logical.

Obvious.

However, evidence may be clouded if the serology is
negative. I have only to be in the presence of symptomatology possibly suggesting the disease, in order to
prescribe praziquantel, the effective medicine. In the
beginning, it was to avoid expenses and other hassles
accompanying the obstinate research protocol advised
by laboratories, as they would suggest various controls
before establishing the final diagnosis.

The result can be surprising: the treatment often frees
patients of recurring urinary infections, which they
have dragged from one urologist to another for years –
forever, if I dare use this arrogant word. On the other

hand, the serology becomes positive, similarly forever, sometimes.

At present, I frequently use this method and obtain the same response.

Here are a few reasons why there is no alternative to taking our four coefficients and their variants, and to adjusting the linear equation at different degrees in order to reach a medical diagnosis.

The base of the polygon is the history of the disease.

This brings a precious contribution when it comes to understanding the disease and deciding whether the usual tactic should be adapted.

But above all, it initiates the study.

If there is no history of disease, then there is no disease to treat, no file to open, no investigation to carry out and no mystery to unveil.

The history of the disease is made manifest in several ways.

Very often, it starts off during travel, a tour, or after a move, or on the sinking sands of a divorce. It appears to be a bout of flu that becomes prolonged.

Or sometimes, more spectacularly, it sets off as encephalitis.

Certain patients develop repeated respiratory infections that sometimes cost them one or more pulmonary biopsies.

Occasionally, the start may be insidious and pass unnoticed.

It can remain so interminably, before capsizing its prey into a world of incoherent dimensions. The trap swallows one down into the hall of mirrors, bewildering mirrors that manage to twist one in simultaneous convexities and concavities, too often causing nose bleeds in the process.

I have several times denounced stress as the triggering factor of diseases.

We meet this tuner of misery in the history of epidemic forms of rickettsia that ravaged different armies made up of undernourished cannon fodder, unprotected against rain and cold.

Let's experience dizziness by contemplating the typhus infecting 25 million Russian soldiers in the First World War and killing three million of them.

Why was this epidemic not present during times of peace?

Our era is generally regarded as a delta with currents that are as strong as the Mississippi.

Apparently, the accumulation of events that have succeeded wartime deaden our senses. Diverse transport mechanisms allow us to zoom over terrestrial and aerial distances. Television, radio and newspapers confront us with catastrophes that defy fiction and force us to contemplate the damage. But are we really without a choice?

Added to this, HIV is a kind of Damocles' sword.

But is it so much more disgusting than the obscure tuberculosis that, before killing Modigliani and his contemporaries by turning them into caverns, left its traces in the bones of Neolithic men and Egyptian mummies?

The chronic form of the condition was considered to be a degenerative or hereditary disease until the end of the 19th century. Laennec, the inventor of the stethoscope, suggested its infectious nature.

Let us contemplate syphilis and its disastrous annihilation. It destroyed Charles VIII and François I, Alexander Borgia and his nephew Caesar Borgia, Toulouse Lautrec, Charles Baudelaire, Alphonse Daudet and Guy de Maupassant, Ivan the Terrible, Henry VIII, and many other geniuses, celebrities and street urchins.

In the 16th century in Paris, it was estimated that a third of the population was contaminated. According to Erasme, all nobles not infected by syphilis were deemed vile and rustic. No need for sexual contact for its contagion: it sufficed to drink from the glass of anyone with a syphilitic lesion on the mouth. During the time of the Tudors, greetings were not made by handshake, but by a kiss on the lips. In the country where I live today, its probably not hygienic caution that makes one say: "Hi, how are you?" followed by "Fine thanks, and you?" — generally continuing on one's way without even a second glance.

Let's go back to pestilence, notably those that accompanied the French and Spanish Inquisitions.

Would you have preferred living during the period of

the medieval wars? In that period, caesarean sections were done at the foot of castles, with so-called knives that were as dirty before being planted into the belly as they were after. This most probably happened among a crowd of onlookers, who screamed louder than the newborn.

If you are still hesitating, I will continue with other suggestions.

I just had a thought for poor Louis XIV, the Sun King, whose body was constantly attacked by fleas, ticks and medical treatments such as bleedings, enemas, scalpels, cauterisation and other nastiness to disinfect his flesh. Remember the' Damned Kings' and the famine of that epoch?

Here is a possible scenario: trenches in the First World War or the guerrilla warfare during World War II.

Let's consider the era prior to anaesthetic. A leg would be amputated on the kitchen table with a dose of alcohol serving as a painkiller and, as a silencer, a cloth was stuffed in the mouth. Eugene Manet, the daring and innovative impressionist, never got over this procedure that was carried out on him at the end of the 19th century.

What fate was one submitted to during that time when antibiotics did not exist? Any microbe was fatal, provided brigands had not already mugged you, and if you were still alive, though sick, the barber exposed you to a chill wind, which was intended to cure you, but brought on double pneumonia. The affair was concluded six feet under ground.

What about life as a Hussar in Napoleons service? During the Russian retreat, if he took refuge in the immense forests, there was the risk of being mauled by a bear or a wolf — providing nothing else had happened during the course of the journey. Alternatively, to escape, he would need to disguise himself in true Stendhal style. Having survived the mournful plains of Waterloo, he must have felt he was facing a kind of 'end of the world'.

More peacefully, an Eskimo has little chance but to become dozy on his ice pack.

And what about "Hiroshima, my love", during and after the atomic bomb in 1945?

Of course, in our day, we are subjected to numerous telephonic assaults. According to Jean Rostand, it requires less for a laboratory rat to develop an experimental ulcer.

Therefore, the future of our gastric and duodenal systems seems quite gloomy. We can only hope that mutations will look after us: a matter of reorganising our carbon material.

They have already rid us of gills and tails. Our brain box has expanded and our apish face has been regulated. Hair on foreheads, hands and feet is no longer paraded by anyone except a few hobbits, a small number of Papuans and other scarce exceptions.

Today, our ears are much too small and should

contain a batch of tympanic membranes all vibrating separately, or at least we should have an extra receptor on top of our heads.

Equally, what can be done with a single tongue to answer all the questions simultaneously hovering around us?

We could also do with four hands to orchestrate our modern world; though feet are no longer strictly necessary.

Of what use is our dentition, other than for having our wisdom teeth removed, garnishing the rest with braces, and for pursuing a war without victory between lead and porcelain? Why so many types of ammunition if we have to give them back anyway?

What is the role of the nose, other than for the red hue it turns when we tell a lie? Truffles are scarce in the under-brush and often germs have no odour.

Contact with the infectious agent may be evident, hidden or forgotten, from a classical tick bite and a set of fleabites, to an unmarked skin.

I remember the anecdote of a doctor from Pietermaritzburg. He claimed to have never been bitten by a tick. It took a few months of treatment to rid him of his amnesia and recognise that the small scar on his right wrist was the sequel of a biopsy done four years previously.

These are the results of the biopsy: cutaneous tumour of 4mm in diameter, origin: insect bite.

Symptomatology constitutes the first side of the polygon.

After an influenza episode, the patient drags along with a fatigue that is as physical as it is mental. The patient endlessly complains of headaches, tenacious headaches resistant to painkillers. They occur often, resembling a constant pressure behind the eyes. If sufferers are not awoken during the night by their intensity, they are present, as consciousness is resumed in the morning. Often they fade away after the patient rises, and then resume vigour in proportion to the nervous stimuli going through the patient.

This situation can be logically explained in the following way: the cranial box, made up of an assembly of bones welded together does not allow any elasticity. Unfortunately, inside this box, some of the capillary's cells are packed with intracellular organisms, which are destroying their protoplasm. These perforated cells are called Foam cells. They suffer from leaks that accumulate, especially at night, when the horizontal position offers insufficient drainage. That is why, after a few moments spent standing, the situation often improves.

Another dubious phenomenon: where have the patients' memories gone?

It is flabbergasting, conversation is impossible, and they forget everything and wander about with paper reminders that go astray at the bottoms of their pockets.

They cannot recall two consecutive numbers. This is a considerable handicap when it comes to dialling a phone number or settling an account. They find it impossible to concentrate.

J R. Radio 702's famous speaker, who makes women's hearts flutter because he has beautiful eyes and we are susceptible, described his brain as being encased in a plastic bag. He could not remember a Trade Union's president's name when he faced him during an interview.

It is a question of the deceleration of mental functions due to the anoxia in which the brain is swamped.

Our intellectual capacities are so clearly dependant on the fluidity of our chemical ingredients. Hard luck.

Chemicals so powerful they have escorted the human race to a holiday on earth. They guide our instincts, give the red colouring to scaly male ostrich feet, command our fantasies, garnish the peacock's crop, modulate the sound of our voices, force salmon to swim up rivers and render us either sublime or beastly. Sometimes very aggressive too.

We owe our fortune, in this case, to our human status. Without this, our fate would be that of stallions, bulls or dogs that are castrated as protection from their ardour.

Chemicals, taking charge of love, strip it of its magic.

And poets sing love songs in poetic chemistry. It is just as beautiful.

It is sometimes in our best interest not to think too much. Reason's implacable medium is not always in favour of our emotions.

Some develop depression, which is sometimes tolerable, and sometimes is not. This originates from the secretion of neurotoxins into our circulation by our damned invaders.

The presence of these neurotoxins can set off psychiatric diseases, such as schizophrenia. Out of nowhere voices converse with you and smells choke you. Whether you will or not, you are projected into the world of apparitions.

Another symptom specific to a schizophrenic, is to feel thoughts and perform actions that have been guided by an external force, often perceived as an extra-terrestrial one. He feels as though he has lost control of the unrolling of his life. The sensation of reality is disturbing and traumatising.

So he takes refuge in a dream with no exit and translates his idle fancies into stereotypical gestures, impulsively generated, the last uniting the next with the help of an invisible string.

Words too are recaptured in an interminable rigmarole, devoid of sense.

For us.

For him, there is no alternative but to maintain this conversation without respite, otherwise panic settles in. The assailant is demanding and reigns supreme. It's like a broken record, endlessly playing the same tune.

Time and again the assailant will make place for silence, maybe even more odious than the gesticulated antics. The nightmare reaches new depths when social living is no longer risked.

In the case of rickettsial schizophrenia, this psychosis is but a symptom of the disease and not the disease itself.

Historically, schizophrenia as a disease remains heterogeneous, which doesn't facilitate its enigmatic origin.

The lives of nine million people could have been saved if Hitler had been treated. His paranoia caused him to perceive society as a huge biological organism. He presented an atypical schizophrenia, like most major affective disorders.

How can they be explained?

How can they be cured?

Generally, one starts by making patients swallow sedatives, stimulants, tranquillisers, euphoric drugs that are supposed to make them change poles.

When they can no longer stand it, or nothing more is unblocked and the family is done complaining, the operating theatre is reserved for the application of electroshocks.

Where is the medical sense in this course of action?

Our professor in Neurology at the University of Louvain, in Belgium, Dr De Reymaker, compared this procedure to one used by certain people to restart a broken alarm clock. They throw it on the floor in the hope of getting it going…

My research on this technique found only that it was applied in the Nazi concentration camps in experiments on Jewish children, and it then entered our medical world, without much further protocol. Apart from statistical studies on its use, I did not come across a scientific publication explaining its physiological mechanism.

It is still used in many countries. With or without the help of straitjackets.

Recently, I treated a farmer suffering from severe fatigue and depression with my antibiotherapy. He had had many sessions of electroshocks during the past couple of years. Before my treatment, he was speechless and almost bedridden. It took me six months to get him back into life, happy and active, but unfortunately, what he said never made sense, and what he did was incomprehensible: his brain had been irreversibly burnt by the electrical power.

Among my patients, I regularly see an occasional victim of this method.

The 'Bolero, brilliant mathematical piece translated in music by Maurice Ravel, was first called: Obsession d'un rythme. It brings the same powerful and convincing theme again and again, louder and louder in a crescendo, with an insistence that becomes physically intolerable. It was also used to shatter the brains of prisoners in concentration camps.

Would the suggestion of experimenting with it as a

treatment for our confused CFS sufferers make any sense?

For both of the above techniques, electroshock and Ravel's Bolero, what could the therapeutic value and the scientific criteria be to warrant their use in CFS patients?

Sometimes, it seems that medicine and law pursue the same achievements, have identical goals and are doing similar jobs. They are just wearing different uniforms, and are claiming different objectives as explanation for their acts.

Against individuals that are definitely ill and dangerous, as well as against convicted criminals, the society's only consideration seems to be its security. Surely, this should only apply to just a minority.

Like goods trains coming from various origins, one should sort out those mental patients in marshalling yards and one would discover that most of them are not more noxious than normal people. By rearranging the wagons according to their cargo, one could compose new trains and send them to new destinations. Not all of them to the dumping yards.

Many of my patients have been the victims of this network, forced to undergo a treatment more than vaguely dangerous, and then confined to a psychiatric hospital.

Thereafter, the aim of the treatment they receive is basically to transform them into zombies, so that the trouble they cause will be shut down.

Never mind the quality of life they are left with, never mind the real reason for their illness. With tablets or injections, no control over life or death is left to them, neither the possibility to choose between the two.

In the name of medicine...

I had better behave or I will be next!

What I could do to dam up the damage would be to change the subject by quoting other medical errors. Such as the way that 'late chlorosis' was treated.

This disease's name is of Greek origin and alludes to the colour of chlorophyll, and it primarily strikes teenage girls. The greenish hue of the skin reflects the serious anaemia from which they are suffering. This condition was treated via bleeding at the beginning of the 20th century. Bleeding was used to treat everything.

The human body was believed to contain 11 to 12 litres of blood. Therefore a bleeding often removed up to three litres of blood, for example in cases of fever, when it was thought that the blood was boiling inside the body and on the verge of producing an explosion.

Generally, bleeding was practiced at the bend of an elbow to start with, and if the response was too slow, another wound was given to the ankle.

Local bleeding was done with the aid of hermaphrodite, aquatic or terrestrial leeches. These were obtainable at the local drugstore — until the Sixties in Europe.

They were conserved in water coming from lakes or rivers, and which was renewed every second day. In this way the optimal concentration of microbes transmitted to the patient during each treatment was certainly obtained.

Puerperal fever could also disturb the medical conscience.

Not so long ago, in obstetric theatres and wards, the doctor transferred to each parturient, without flinching, murderous streptococci adhering to the cuffs of his white jacket.

But enough said about iatrogenic diseases. Even if errors of the past often give perspective on today's torments, I only needed a moment's digression.

Carpe diem.

CFS is on the menu, or more precisely its diagnosis.

Before losing our way, we were busy describing its symptoms.

Fatigued patients very often present with night sweats, reflecting their state of inflammation. They awake in the middle of the night, with their hair clinging to their foreheads, looking as haggard and wet as if they had just crossed a river dragging a few rotten fish. It is this particular odour caused by the sweats that they have to integrate into their daily lives thereafter.

Their eyes become red and dry, are irritated, and roll around in their orbits. In addition to this, light sets off an untoward burning sensation that can no longer bring tears to their eyes. Ophthalmic drops become part of their obsessions, trying not to lose them is another matter.

Throats feel forever scratchy, as if they had swallowed too many frogs.

Ears start buzzing and even whistling, on a relentless shrill note. How frustrating. Sound can be painful. How overburdened they are. They are instantly recognisable: on entering a room, they immediately throw themselves on the Hi-fi to turn it off before even greeting you. Even, the most sophisticated use plastic cutlery, to avoid the grating of metal on their plates.

In the abdomen, a tenacious throb takes up its domicile, and after a few days concentrates in the area below and to the right of the navel. Many medical files and abdomens will be opened, and many therapeutic routes will be explored because of the pain.

Often, the CFS candidate complains of serious muscular pains, without having done vigorous exercise or having been beaten up.

Joints are also a problem and become swollen, distended by fluid. In some cases, the joints take on a marbled, violet colour of almost corpse-like lividity. However, the origin is the same: a lack of blood circulation in the blood vessels.

Some articulations remain permanently deformed, and will drive the sufferers to the next stop: the rheumatologist. He will prescribe what I do not like and what you have probably guessed: the ubiquitous cortisone.

Lately, I have seen a patient in his early sixties who was aching all over. Plus, he was tired.

The doctor that he had consulted before me had comforted him by reminding him of his age and his frequent motorbike accidents. Indeed, he had broken a few bones in this way.

Had I played along with my colleague's opinion, I would not have tested him, but he insisted on a feeling of heaviness and exhaustion. Perhaps I was also hoping to find a person who was not sick.

This man's biology showed evidence of a series of infections. There were five different strains – rickettsia, mycoplasma and bilharzias — and his white blood cells were grossly depleted.

I saw him again recently. His aches have disappeared and he's bursting with dynamism. In parallel, his white blood cells have revived. Six months of treatment was enough to change the course of his life.

After a period of illness, new symptoms become apparent.

Vision is blurred due to a lack of focus, black dots or yellow-orange rings float in the field of vision, without having inevitably to develop multiple sclerosis.

Defeat should be admitted after having bought all the spectacles on the market.

My father finished his life practically blind, by virtue of accumulating inflammations of the uvea, due to the splashes of rickettsial antigens in the conjunctiva.

I knew a patient who woke up one day seeing only in black and white in the right eye. I sent her for a scan. A tumour of the optic nerve, one centimetre in diameter, could be outlined. The ophthalmic surgeon suggested removing the eye. I wanted to start with a gentler technique: tetracycline. Her tumour pulverised.

People suffering from chronic fatigue commonly experience a cold sensation in the hands and feet, and sometimes at the level of the ears and nose. This is what is called Raynaud's syndrome. I have seen hands of such a vivid violet that they cannot go unnoticed, even by quite colour-blind people.

Hands that come to mind belong to a young girl with a pretty face, which lights up in a toothless smile as she describes her sheep grazing on the Karoo plains. She had seen numerous doctors who had applied different treatments, among others total tooth extraction for recalcitrant pains of the gums.

I have seen other hands that resembled tufts of ice cream, going from red to yellow and finishing in purple.

Our receiver develops easy haematomas, due to a vascular system that is too fragile. I think of a woman whose legs have been covered in bruises for a number of years. Her bruises fade at each treatment.

Neurological symptoms take longer to appear and the diagnosis of multiple sclerosis or other neurological diseases can only be specified after several years. If it is specified.

Our patient may also have cardiac pains and suffer from shortness of breath, and have palpitations that are sometimes frightening. This gives one the opportunity of applying the theatrical Valsalva manoeuvre. This consists of firmly applying both thumbs to the eyes of the person suffering from tachycardia, and deeply massaging the ocular globe. This leads to a vagal reaction, in other words an instant and spectacular deceleration of the cardiac rhythm, leaving the patient struck dumb with admiration.

Others suddenly develop allergies that were foreign to them. They awake with eyelids that are so swollen they seem to be joined, and skin covered in geographical maps set in relief, salmon-coloured and horribly itchy, that appear and disappear, often according to temperature.

I sometimes come across allergies so severe that they mask the rest of the symptomatology.

Diets omitting flour and yeast are fastidious and offer little help. Antihistamines render them even sleepier, those who already feel as though they are under premedication. Because, ever dominant in the picture, one will find fatigue.

Fatigue.
Magisterially vindictive, it commands an urgency that is as great as hunger can be. It commands the present moment, impetuous and sovereign, like a physical and

mental hypoglycaemia of sorts.

It is cellular anoxia's signature due to the presence of micro-organisms in the cells' cytoplasm.

It condemns its victims to a tough life.

It becomes difficult for them to get up in the morning. They buy themselves several alarm clocks and set them all off at the same time.

They fall asleep at the wheel, provided they are still able to drive.

Their professional life is affected. Even for the strong stud, making love becomes drudgery, impossible in the morning and certainly not at night. Soon this pleasure, still risked certain Saturday or Sunday afternoons, become unattainable.

They shift around so as not to lose sight of chair or bed, wherever they may be.

Children are forced to abandon school. University students cut short their studies. Adults become incapable of maintaining their positions at work and their services are soon terminated, if not by management, by their own initiative.

They often need to carefully follow the state of their finances.

Their social lives wither away. They lose friends that have tired of hearing them complain, though they may no longer have the energy for even that.

Where can one find the energy to do anything but out of vital necessity?

Everything puts them in a state. They have long

abandoned hanging out the washing. By this stage, they have renounced combing their hair, as it is too difficult to raise an arm for even a few seconds.

They are forced to learn to save energy.

Do not hold it against them if they do not answer your questions. It is not that they do not like you or are being impolite, but rather that they no longer know what to say, as their brains have become fuddled, and even if they did still function, their tongues would become the culprits, being doughy from fatigue.

They can sleep for up to 24 hours at a stretch without feeling rested.

They gulp down phenomenal quantities of coffee. But did not Red Bull work well yesterday?

Nothing works, nothing, nothing except that hole as big and as black as the night to where the disease is driving them.

Their medical cabinet becomes laden with vitamins, which have no real success. They are deemed to be depressed sloths. But then, they are rather depressed at being tired.

This horse must be cared for, and the fridge must be filled, and the car does not start anymore and life is an abyss.

What energy they have left does not even allow them to cry out, and anyway, we could not care less about the vastness of their calamity.

Too bad, sighs our chronic fatigue sufferer as he

laboriously turns over in bed, after having renounced opening his eyelids. Too heavy.

He becomes engulfed by a slumber that is more reminiscent of a coma. Sometimes he remains so for countless days, abandoned by anything labelled life, in a state of stupor, as is met with … cases of typhus

It is not easy to die on this earth.

The thief has nicked it all: from magnesium, sugar, oxygen, friends, work, and money, thinking capacity, until the simple energy to get up.

And that's not all.

Because after the fatigue that is as paralysing as an anaesthetic, there is the one that keeps you awake, whether you like it or not.

This is called manic-depression. It scoffs at sedatives and narcotics, straight jackets and electric shocks. It runs through your veins, shakes your body in its own crazy rhythm.

It is as tangible as stupor, as unconquerable as hurt, as organic as sweat.

Only it is more vicious, more extravagant.

So if you have reached this stage, and nobody comes to your aid, don't worry, you have won the game of the goose, the next visitor will finally bring the solution. It will erase everything, up to the shadow of your body.

Its name is death.

Sometimes it plays coyly.

Is this what you are waiting for?

If the answer is no, one of my patients gave me advice

for those days of desperation. When he felt suicidal, he phoned me to ask for a prescription of tetracycline. According to him, this was the best antidepressant. He is not here to confirm this, as he committed suicide without leaving a note.

That is why, in the name of all my people, I ask your help in my anti-rickettsial campaign.

The clinical examination is the third side of the polygon.

It is a confirmation of the patient's symptoms and often discloses similar pointers from one patient to another.

The very distinctive pallor of the face resembles the colour of cement, a greyish yellow. This is another indication of insufficient blood and oxygen circulation in the superficial blood capillaries. The return of a fresh tone is generally one of the first changes established during the course of the treatment.

Peripheral vascularisation is poor, pulses are, sometimes, not palpable.

Their eyes are bloodshot with dilated capillaries and tearing is rare, resembling a prelude to Sjögren's disease. In the evolution of the latter, the tongue becomes equally dry, hindering speech and swallowing.

The inflamed throat appears bright red, sometimes with white spots. Most patients do not complain about it as the tissue only becomes tender when it is in the process of being distended.

The ganglions grow in size and become sensitive to palpation. They are found in the neck, under the arms, and in the groin. These are sometimes subject to a biopsy, which probably will only highlight the presence of inflamed tissue. The fistula accompanying the process of healing will almost certainly never completely close.

One of every two hearts examined presents anomalies. The auscultation reveals a murmur, a click, a tachycardia or an arrhythmia, which will leave the patient panic-stricken. The cardiologist confirms the anomaly and reassures the patient. The present pathology is qualified to be 'innocent'. Why should one ask questions when confronted with innocence?

Splenomegaly is more rarely found. Generally, one who presents a large spleen gets rid of it quite quickly.

In the great majority of cases, the right iliac fossa is sensitive to palpation, and can even be sore.

The liver is often enlarged and occasionally tender.

Neurological signs such as loss of sensitivity, loss of reflexes, loss of muscle tone or muscle mass are notice-able now and then.

Dermatological anomalies are frequent and varied, going from eczema to psoriasis, super pigmentations to ulcers, from a giant urticaria to dermographism. The last mentioned example will allow you to imprint for a few instants, the patient's name or other letters, upon their bellies preferably, using the back of the nail.

Joints will sometimes be deformed. When they are,

they may be discreetly so or considerably, momentary or permanent.

Clinical biology completes our polygon.

The following tests systematically apply to each patient.

On the whole, the blood tests place emphasis on the white blood cells, habitually heightened in the active phase and diminished towards the end of the disease's evolution. The blood platelets are often lowered. Simultaneously, a slight case of anaemia is perceived.

The sedimentation rate is usually raised.

The study of iron frequently uncovers a plunge in the percentage saturation.

An elevation of the iron levels bears witness to the state of inflammation of the surroundings.

The infectious agents also threaten the sugar level. This is especially obvious in cases of diabetes, which were well controlled before the arrival of the CFS.

Studies of hepatic function show anomalies in 70% of cases. Investigation for glandular fever is performed where this applies.

Studies of renal function do not seem to be directly influenced by the infection.

The same goes for thyroid function. However, thyroid antibodies are readily elevated.

Auto-immune factors, such as Protein C Reactive, the Antinuclear Factor and the Rheumatoid Factor are regularly disturbed. This is so even in cases where rheumatoid symptomatology is silent.

In cases where cancer is suspected, the specific markers are scanned.

HIV testing is carried out if necessary.

To this, investigations of curable infections are added.

More specifically, this includes the detection of antibody levels against five different rickettsial antigens, four different chlamydia antigens, one mycoplasma, as well as the schistosome antibodies against bilharzia for patients who have been in Africa.

To bring the rickettsial antibody levels to light, we resort to Giroud's Micro-agglutination test, for which we employ the following antigens:

● Rickettsia prowazeki, which is the epidemic form of typhus, and has always been present in the history of humanity.

● Rickettsia mooseri, which is supposedly endemic.

● Rickettsia conori, which is responsible for tick bite fever, belonging to the spotted fever group.

● Coxiella Burnetti, which is commonly known as Q fever.

Specific strains of rickettsial antigens are directly collected from the bowels of infected ticks and other arthropods. They are then pulverized. This mixture is then homogenised and injected into the peritoneal cavity of the guinea pig, mouse, hamster, rabbit or fertilised eggs, to be cultivated.

The suspension of antigens destined for the study of

antibodies is placed in a diluted solution of formol to attenuate its virulence.

A drop of the patient's serum is added to a drop of diluted known antigen solution, on a slide. The two drops are mixed. Known antigens are used to detect the presence of unidentified antibodies and will react against them by agglutination. The slide is dried, and then dyed and dried again before it is read microscopically.

Agglutination occurs or it does not. It is not a question of personal interpretation. Test quality depends on antigen quality.

In time, variation of the curve of antibodies often reveals the reactivation of dormant foci. In other words the presence of a chronic active infection. One refers to it as a 'see saw'.

In cases where the test gives negative results and where the symptoms suggest the disease, it could be interesting to repeat the test to detect a possible fluctuation in the antibodies' level.

Tests can give a negative reading if patients are being or have been treated with cortisone.

As for any infections and as expected, positive tests can emanate from people who display no symptoms (Giroud, Jadin; 26% according to Drancourt).

As Paul Giroud concluded in the Bulletin de la société de pathologie exotique in 1963: "Of all the given data, the imperative value of the antibodies level, conceived in the laboratory, stands out. It does not resist logic or clinical concepts, but concerning its indicatory value, Micro-agglutination remains extremely useful when used in conjunction with clinical signs."

Comparative studies between the Immuno-fluorescence test, the ELISA test, and the Micro-agglutination test were performed in Professor JB Jadin's laboratory. Similar results were obtained.

In October 1997, as mentioned before, the Brumpt prize of the Pasteur Institute of Paris was awarded to my father for his work on rickettsia.

The test is simple, reliable and specific when valid antigens are at hand.

Another reason for my applying this test is because from a very young age I have been familiar with it.

The last logical reason is simply that we do not yet employ any other routine tests for the detection of specific rickettsial antibodies, against the different strains currently in South Africa. This is why this technique remains our choice in today's circumstances.

Our second objective in the search for curable infections points to chlamydias.

These are the four antigens participating in the diagnosis:

- Chlamydia Q18, which falls into the neo-rickettsial group and is the cause of many infertility problems and abortions in sheep, as my father has reported in his formularies of biological results.

For women, the same germ could precipitate the same result. Nevertheless gynaecologists used to hold stress responsible for the last example. Should one conclude that sheep have no stress in their lives and women no chlamydias? The Micro-agglutination is equally used to detect it.

- Chlamydia pneumonia, the origin of recurrent chest infections.
- Chlamydia psittaci, transmitted, as its name indicates, by contact with parrots and other birds.
- Chlamydia trachomatis, identified in all age groups of the population, although it is considered as a sexually transmitted disease. When this type of chlamydia is diagnosed in young children, the parents tested for the same germ are found to be negative.

Our third investigation into the infections is directed against mycoplasmas.

The antigen Mycoplasma pneumonia is the only one available in South African laboratories today.

For our last routine investigation, the detection of bilharzia, as well as for Chlamydia pneumoniae, trachomatis and psittaci, and for mycoplasma, we resort to Dr LVR. Laboratories, where the method of Immunofluorescence has been used since the year 2000. More recently, he has introduced the use of this very technique for detection of Coxiella burnetti.

This allows us to compare the results of both laboratories, which are generally confirmed.

The biological investigation has a double purpose.

Not only does it have to indirectly bring the germ's presence to light, but also allows us to determine whether the germ is alive and aggressive at the various levels of different human organs. Without these complementary tests, we would be forced to study the seesaw's evolution of the patient's antibodies. Mission impossible.

All the possible parasites that man could serve as host are not necessarily in the active phase at the time of the blood test. How can one find out if they are dead or dormant?

Differentiating antibodies into two groups is not a great help.

IgMs are supposed to identify present infections, and IgGs old infections. This conclusion is clear theoretically, but contradicted when put into practice.

In fact, if their assemblies are traced in the serum of patients submitted to antibiotic treatment, a fluctuation is observed in both groups, particularly in the second.

Man and his parasites form an ecosystem managed by numerous factors, which will influence the results of the blood test.

● the patient's age should be taken into consideration when interpreting the test; as the number of people presenting positive serology increases with age, but the quality diminishes with age;

- past and present environment should also be taken into account, as demonstrated in the anecdote of the farmer and his brother;
- the associated presence of bacteria, viruses and other parasites;
- physical activity may also influence the state of the immune system;
- similarly nutrition, vitamin intake and the intake of drugs such as anti-inflammatories, antibiotics, or cortisone that paralyse the immune system as already mentioned;
- diverse traumas
- also the time of year and time of day, which could cause an oscillation in the pendulum of the production of antibodies.

Thus as time and patients have gone by, we have become incapable of establishing a valid diagnosis in the absence of our four points.

Here is a practical example: It's not the blood test, nor the history of disease, nor even the patient's symptoms that lead me to deduce an inflammation at heart level or at the level of the right iliac depression. In the same light, I will not find the elevation of the level of thyroid antibodies from the symptoms or the clinical examination. In the same way, the level of antibodies for epidemic typhus will not tell me how many glasses of fresh milk the patient drinks a day. Nor will the clinical examination help me understand why this patient, though so ill, does not present with more than a weak level of antibodies.

The use of my polygon has given me access to a diagnostic method based on the most classical teachings of medicine.

I have recaptured my pastoral heritage and prudently left new approaches aside.

I have no understanding of iridology, reflexology, the use of pendulums, examinations in practical laboratories done on fresh blood that bring to mind images as fantastical as those in Star Wars, procedures that are balanced on a computer screen, the analysis of hair to reveal your varied deficiencies, etc.

The use of these daring procedures would make me lose my balance.

After establishing a diagnosis using sufficiently qualified laboratories, I put into effect a treatment that is renowned for is efficiency and available in conventional pharmacies.

What could be more boringly traditional?

Yet, in South Africa's medical world, I am labelled as controversial, and my methods are judged to be experimental.

I hope the expression suggested by my dear Penny Forbes: "You'll be damned if you do and you'll be damned if you don't" won't apply in my case.

CHAPTER 12:

THE TREATMENT

"Non-proven statements are only coincidences."
—*La logique ou l'art de raisonner par*
Y. Demas-Rigoutsos et R. Lalement—

It does the diagnosis justice. It pushed me into writing this book. Because it does exist. Within the reach of hands, wallets and stomachs.

In addition to this, as it is no longer very youthful, it is of proven safety and efficacity.

It releases those on the rack, makes the paralysed walk, rids the possessed of demons, gives sight to the blind and breath to the exhausted. Some find it miraculous.

But it is a medical treatment.

Not a game of poker, its application relies on empiricism dating far back and is determined by the structure of the infectious agents and by the damage they cause to the human body as a whole.

The treatment of the syndrome of chronic fatigue aims at eliminating the infectious factors accompanying this state, without lingering on the symptoms escorting it.

First of all, a list of the germs must be established, no matter if incomplete, so long as to be focused on those that we are pharmaceutically equipped to deal with.

For the quality of existence to rise like a hot-air balloon, it is often enough to release ballast.

The body, once free of its hoard of parasites, will regain primary integrity of its functions with scar tissue as its only limitation.

How can this mission be accomplished?

How can the survival and reproduction of these foreign bodies be prevented within our bodies?

If they find us seductive, it is not because of our charming eyes. It is because the makeup of our protoplasm looks to the invader like the Promised Land. So, mouths watering at our blood, attacking our membranes, using their chemistry to penetrate our physique, they transform the whole into a conquered land.

— And as if to dislodge them, the conquered land was changed by bartering the contents of its protoplasm?

— Okay, but how can this be practically achieved without changing the nature of the human tissue?

— By taking vitamins for instance, or supplements, or any odd minerals as well as proteins.

— This would undoubtedly enrich us, rendering us more desirable than the average Petri dishes, which are the ones designed to grow germs in laboratories.

There was once a lovely garden filled with a variety of vegetations. The ravishing flowers were sadly suffocated by heaps of weeds. The owner, aware of the situation, flooded his garden with fertilizers, hoping to strengthen his flowers. The result was disastrous. He was not a good gardener.

To solve the problem, should he not first have eliminated the weeds instead of feeding them?

The answer is obvious — it would more difficult if the questions were in the form of multiple choices.

— How absurd!

Let's find something else: a prototype for a balanced diet to optimise our different functions, antioxidants for protection against free radicals. Rectifying an imbalance cannot be destructive, or complicated to achieve with our physiological knowledge of the human body.

— The difficulty does not lie so much in our knowledge, as in the lack of data.

What we are sure of on the surface may be an inverted image at greater depth. Or maybe not.

— Before repairing our metabolism, should we not rather try to shorten the intruders' stay?

Do away with what they are waiting for open-mouthed, all fangs revealed, asphyxiating us with their malevolent endotoxins. Cease the production of ATP, close the sugar tap and cut down the energy level to forbid the prolongation of their stratagems.

If they are not given what they came for, they will leave the Noah's Ark of our bodies or ultimately perish. Unshakable logic. Even the most sedentary and narrow-minded would react.

— So, let's give it a bash. The first step is to put our metabolism into hibernation, followed by the second, which is the starvation of the unwelcome.

— Could it be a question of an iatrogenic hallucination, taking patients for marmots?

— No, it is a method exploiting the fact that our metabolism is largely perfected, when compared with those of the infinitely tiny.

If we stop eating, they are slowed down, pass through a period of fasting, and we will not need to commence our famine phase to see them starve from theirs. Fasting could rid us of morbid substances, and substances not unwholesome for all, which have invaded our bodies with time.

Thus, not only the intracellular organisms are deprived of their share of nutritional elements indispensable to their vital functions. However, they are also forced to leave the cytoplasm, because the latter decomposes after a certain duration of fasting, as Dr M Kunde proved, subsequent to conducting involved studies on the physiological mechanism of fasting at the University of Chicago from 1923. He explains that when bodyweight is reduced by about 45%, then restored to the original weight by a normal diet, the restoration will be composed of new protoplasm. In this way, dormant rickettsiae that are nestled in the heart of our cytoplasm, which forms part of the same protoplasm, are evacuated. Fasting eliminates the contents as well as the container, before re-establishing the latter.

The conquered land will be assisting to the death of a number of its cells, some by necrosis, resulting from the acute injury of starving, and others by entering apoptosis. This means in Greek 'fall of the leaves'. It is a mechanism programming the death of cells. The mechanism can be activating by internal and external signals. This applies concurrently to the invaders.

Even if the weight loss does not achieve the required percentage for protoplasm wastage, the parasites are plunged into a period of merciless famine.

In the meanwhile, we are breaking the short phase of gluconeogenesis, during which our bodies use their proteins to maintain a minimal blood sugar level.

We are then branched into a system that allows us to consume our own adipose tissue, vulgarly named 'fats', as a primary energy source.

250

In my clinical observations, patients who have carried out a period of fasting generally felt better.

How many historical celebrities can we quote, who have been examples? Socrates followed by his disciple Plato, Jesus and Moses prior to him, Pythagoras, Mohammed, Buddha and Ghandi.

After them entire nations did the same. For different reasons, ranging from religion, politics, power, acts of protest or even health reasons.

In fact, in prehistoric times, fasting was inevitable. Our ancestors were not acquainted with shopping centres, fires, refrigerators or tin cans. They lived in a wilderness where they had to forage for herbs, fruit, insects or larger animals in order to survive.

Of course, they were familiar with hunger.

It was part of their era's contingencies.

In our day, the crocodile feeds once a week and stows its leftovers, rather than swallow them as soon as its stomach hollows. The same goes for our neighbours the lions, found in the little nature reserve a few kilometres from our home, as well as all other lions on earth and many other wild animals.

The bear watches indifferently as potential prey files past when winter gets rough. What pushes it to hibernation? Is it a matter of a survival mechanism that forms part of its genetic heritage?

A mechanism forgotten by man, too evolved to

question the memory of ancestral predominance. Who is interested in the cave man's fasting?

And what if fasting, not famine, were a defence mechanism against infectious agents that may invade our bodies, less equipped for the storage of provisions than we are, as a sort of natural protection against the growth of diseases in the long term?

Hippocrates, a father figure, said: "In nourishing the diseased, the disease is nourished."

Equally, animals stop eating when they are sick.

Instinct rids them of their appetite.

And us, what does it have to say, our instinct? Would we listen if it suggested a less automatic provisioning?

Like the Pygmies who blissfully digest their monthly elephant.

Like the Bushmen, a proud and joyful people, whose gods stay in place as long as ancestral traditions are maintained, notably that of eating only a few times a month, without knowing why, if not for the physical well being that flows from it.

Although specialists in fasting do not advise it in cases of tuberculosis, cancer, or leprosy, its proper place in the treatment of rickettsia has not been outlined yet. For instance, some patients use it as a last resort. Others use it more regularly as a means of detoxification. Our experience in the matter is in its early stages.

The treatment that I use and have been refining over the past 10 years consists mainly of a pulsed and regular therapy of certain tetracyclines. Their use is alternated and combined. It is never prescribed in a continuum or at low dosage.

As mentioned above, rickettsiae reproduce intracellularly. They reproduce until the cell explodes. This takes about a month. They are then tipped out into the bloodstream where they cannot survive. So cellular intrusion is once more in focus, rickettsia mature, ready for binary fission and the second offensive ballet.

It is at this point of their development that we find ourselves after administering the first antibiotic treatment. The treatment has emptied the cell of its contents without waiting for the necessary distension of the membrane. Empirically, it determines the start of the cellular cycle. Pragmatically the counter is set at zero.

Then we simply have to apply the antibiotherapy in rhythm with the target's regular development, for a length of seven to 10 days.

Many patients clearly illustrate this phenomenon. In fact, the majority present a renewed outbreak of their symptoms towards the end of the three weeks interval between treatments.

An obvious example is that of a little boy whose big green eyes dominated his gentle face, while his frail body was dissipating under the hold of a multitude of parasites.

He was first diagnosed as suffering from an atypical muscular dystrophy, of a vaguely genetic origin, and after being subjected to a few inconclusive pulmonary biopsies, he was pumped with cortisone. As a result, he went from 30 to 50 kilograms and did not complain of pain anymore. The parents, who were confused, stopped the treatment.

The little patient lost weight and his joints started to swell again. Out of desperation, the parents settled an appointment with my receptionist.

The first time I saw him, he could hardly walk, was groaning with pain and covered with sweat. His knees were enormous and marbled, and the patella was knocking the femur like ice in water. A few toes and fingers were violaceous. His heart was beating wildly.

After discovering a strong multi-infectious condition accompanying his auto-immune factors, antibio-therapy was given to him for more than a year.

At each treatment, the joints' volume would reduce, as pain and fever would vanish. It took exactly 72 hours to reach this result. But three weeks later, the pathology reappeared. Despite the recurrence, symptoms did not present with the same severity as before. His condition clearly improved. He went back to school and lived a happy live.

As his brother had dental cavities, he accompanied him on a visit to the dentist. The practitioner empha-sised the dangers of tetracyclines to dental tissue. He maintained that he would lose teeth if he carried on with this regime. The parents, alarmed by this comment and probably tired of the regular relapses, stopped consulting me.

After a few months, he came back as an emergency. His abdomen was distended by a large quantity of liquid. With the help of the radiologist, I soon excluded any cancerous origin. Following this, an abdominal aspiration was necessary to analyse the nature of this ascitis. Therefore, I referred him to a paediatric colleague. However, he did not follow my suggestion. Instead, he dried the sick abdomen with a potent diuretic and decided to search in his books for the diagnosis. He pointed out the list of different causes of ascitis in children, on page 1 229 from Nelson, a paediatric manual, while discussing our patient's case. With relief I quickly spotted the words schistosomiasis (bilharzia) and chlamydia amongst the infectious agents responsible for ascitis.

"According to our investigations, this ascitis does not originate from the liver," he commented. " His liver function is about normal and the abdominal scan does not show anything. The same applies to his kidneys. It is not of cardiac origin, as I asked a cardiologist to check it out. It is not infectious," he carried on, "there is no cancer, no renal, nor pancreatic tumour. This must fall under this column", he showed me referring to the section 'miscellaneous'. "This means that we are in the presence of an auto-immune disease," he concluded with confidence.

"But why not infectious? Did you see the results of your laboratory requisition concerning chlamydia and bilharzia? It shows a high positivity," I did wonder pointing out the child's tests.

"Impossible," he retorted. "You treated him for those infections over a long period of time. Therefore he must be free of them. Regarding bilharzia, this very clean little boy does not play in dirty water. We are facing here a false positivity. Let us not waste time. You will see him improving on cortisone."

I then phoned Dr LVR, the pathologist. "No, I guarantee you, there is no cross-reaction between chlamydia and schistosomiasis antibodies and auto-immune factors. Send me a specimen of this fluid for confirmation."

In a last attempt at dialogue with the paediatrician, he settled the discussion: "Really, you have a lot of admira-tion for your father."

The ascitis' aspiration never took place.

At 10 years of age, my little patient put back his excess kilos. Tragedies at all times display the same pacifying atmosphere of finality by closing the door on hope. It somehow reassures and everybody is happy.

Except me.

When he was under my care, I introduced him to the daughter of my domestic helper, P, who was 30 years old and radiant with health. Their medical histories were similar and I thought that way I could encourage the parents of my young patient.

Five years earlier, P had suffered bouts of high fever and rheumatic aches with severe weight loss.

Convinced she was suffering from AIDS, she left our residence to go and die somewhere else. When I found out what it was all about, I begged her mother to ask her to come back. She eventually agreed. She was not to be recognised. Wide-open eyes in a wasted body were looking at the beyond. Lots of dying people are like that. All that was left of her were distended knees full of fluid and emaciated witch-like hands.

The blood collection was difficult because the veins collapsed as soon as they were in contact with the needle. In the corner of the room, her mother and her one-year-old daughter were waiting on events, submissive after centuries of accepting fate.

The results were not long in coming: HIV was non-reactive.

Then hope returned. The next blood collection, although as difficult as the first one, did not smell of the death sentence. My science recovered its sense and the investigations confirmed positivity for R+ C+ M+ B+ all auto-immune factors and a deficiency of iron and white cells.

Her treatment, seven days of tetracyclines per month, was immediately started and lasted for three years.

She recovered, with the same picture of undulating symptoms close to the ascendant and oblique lines representing the progress of the disease. Only three months of treatment were necessary for her to walk, six months to carry her baby on her back, and one year to open tins. Now she manages to work and to dance.

Her residual lordosis emphasises her buttocks back in callipygian shape, her knees do not simplify the legs' pattern and her hands are still slightly deformed. The sound of laughter testifies to the joy of good health and the continuing whiteness of her teeth could be an advertisement for tetracyclines.

I advised her to take at least three weeks of antibiotics per year for the rest of her life. This is to prevent damage caused by a possible reawakening of small infectious nests.

Not only is the pulse therapy used to match the rickettsial development cycle, but by doing so, the build up of resistance by the microbes against antibiotics is minimised.

Resistance to the antibiotic very often occurs when their administration is continuous, mainly at a low dosage, and when they are given alone, as described by Giroud.

This is the situation we have when treating acne and malaria. In those cases, doxycyclines or minocyclines are prescribed at a minimum dosage for months. Acne will disappear, malaria will be more or less controlled, but what will happen to the patient the day he develops an intracellular infection?

This is why, we are in favour of the formula 'maximum dosage of tetracycline, meeting the highest concentration in the plasma and in the limit of gastric tolerance, preferably given in association with other antibiotics' recommended by P Giroud and H Floch.

When antibiotics are administered continuously at a high dosage, not many germs will survive their use. But the few that are mutating may give birth to a new generation of super-bugs, which would soon be a world catastrophe.

A biological nightmare costing years of work and loss of human lives.

Another advantage of the pulse antibiotherapy is the resting periods given to the consumer's body, trying to get rid of the toxins produced by the dying germs and the damaged tissues, to resettle into a certain shape before the next attack.

The high dosage is of course kept within the limits of safety.

Goodman et al highlights permanent liver damage following intravenous administration of tetracyclines. Therefore, this method has to be avoided with almost no exception.

Liver damage has not been reported after the use of oral therapy, except in the presence of renal failure or pregnancy. Those two conditions have to be excluded before starting treatment.

In our daily experience of oral administration of tetracyclines, the liver function tests, if normal to start with, will stay normal. If they are abnormal before the oral intake of our treatment, they will improve during therapy and in most cases return to perfect normality. Cases of fatty acid depots, as shown by liver scan, before and after six months to one year of treatment, have disappeared (1 MS, 4 CFS). This confirms the well-documented fact that rickettsia- like agents are far more hepato-toxic than tetracyclines.

The tolerance of the patient is also a factor that we cannot ignore in the practical administration of the treatment. We will have to consider the gastric toler- ance and the general tolerance.

The gastric intolerance is not often severe enough to force us to interrupt the treatment, especially if the patient uses a gastric protector such as a proton pump inhibitor and takes his medication on a full stomach. Should it still happen, it will generally be successfully prevented by doubling the dosage of the proton pump inhibitor during the administration of the antibiotics, and if necessary, the use of the gastric pump inhibitor can be extended before and after the administration of the tetracyclines, after which gastric problems are rare.

The general tolerance of the treatment is directly related to the Jarisch Herxheimer reaction (HR), which is a reactivation of old symptoms and/or exacer- bation of present symptoms that occur while patients are taking antibiotherapy.

It is much more unpleasant and much more frequent than the gastric intolerance. Patients often think this is flu. Headaches might be severe, sometimes accompa- nied by rigors and fever. At times, the blood pressure rises, followed by a fall to near shocks levels. To weaken its severity, acetaminophen can be given.

Some may feel like they're dying, but this does not

usually last.

Its manifestation has a very important diagnostic and prognostic value. It means that the antibiotics are reaching their target, and it is due to the release of the dying microbes into the blood circulation.

It may or may not parallel a serological reactivation, showing an increase of the antibody level in the blood. Indeed, as the antibiotics are ridding the germs from the cells to throw them back into the circulation, the immune system, in the presence of their multitude, will be stimulated, just as should happen when homeopathic medications are taken.

The difference lies in the origin of the antigens: they come from your own body if you are swallowing antibiotics, but they are added into your system in the case of homeopathic remedies.

The HR will fade with the number of treatments received, as will the number of germs. It is generally only the first three treatments that will produce serious discomfort.

This type of reaction is similar to the one occurring when penicillin is given in the presence of syphilis. The administration of penicillin to syphilitic patients will be followed by the release of a massive amount of treponemas into the blood stream, which will generate a systemic response. The reaction that this phenomenon creates has killed many patients and stayed unexplained for a long time. Those patients were not allergic to penicillin. Why should it be fatal?

Herxheimer came up with this brilliant explanation: it was the crowd of treponemas dying in the blood stream that was responsible for the shock and the death of the patient. By systematically using the probenecid in case of severe syphilis, the patients were saved.

The tetracyclines are alternated for of many reasons.

One important reason is that a patient is practically always infected with many strains of rickettsiae, mycoplasma and chlamydia, which have different sensitivities to the various tetracyclines or combinations. Although this fact is quite difficult to establish in vitro, it is quite clear in our clinical experience.

We also use the antibiotics alternatively, because we are concerned that if we keep administrating the same antibiotic for a prolonged period of time, even though in a resting period, the parasite might build resistance to it and this would be the end of the efficiency of the treatment.

A colleague of mine has illustrated this fact. As he initially obtained excellent results with the use of a particular doxycycline, he stuck to it for a while and wondered about the absence of a further good response, until we together analysed the reason of this absence of further progress.

Another reason to rotate the use of tetracyclines, is that patients show individual sensitivity to different tetracyclines or combinations of it, and there is very often an exclusive reaction to a specific treatment.

Indeed patients are genetically coded with different pools of binding receptor proteins. The particular treatment of choice for each individual can then be used preferentially, especially when a short course will do, as in cases of relapses.

Tetracyclines are combined with quinolones, macrolides or metronidazole, because rickettsiae, chlamydia and mycoplasma present a wide heterogeneity of susceptibility to different drugs.

During a congress on CFS, a colleague, who was upset by the use of quinolones, approached me. To him, by doing so, I was in contradiction with my diagnosis of rickettsial infections, because quinolones are supposed to treat something else.

It was as though I was hiding something, and that put my integrity in question, despite the fact of my success.

Once again, I am amazed that all over the world, one will always find someone to criticise my method, but the clinical successes I obtain using these specific methods do not seem to be subject to the same interest.

The treatment will often need to be prolonged.

Again, there are many reasons for it. First, by nature, the germ shows a slow evolution profile in which some foci are dormant, encapsulated and therefore protected from antibiotherapy. Others are actively multiplying in the cytoplasm of the cells of their host, and therefore can be treated. The dormant forms have to become active to enable us to treat them.

There are multiple foci of rickettsiae, all lying around, in different parts of our bodies, with a different look: young, successful, dividing and invasive, or quiet, slow and captive in a vacuole.

Another reason to extend the treatment lies in the fact that each treatment will help the immune system to produce and maintain a proper and efficient level of antibodies, as explained above. This theory can be read in Legag's work.

The length of the disease should logically imply a prolonged treatment. In our experience, this point is not always true. Patients, ill for many years, may recover after a few months of treatment; just as patients presenting with a short period of illness might take months, even years to recover. The explanation for this could be that many co-factors of this condition are still unknown. If we face a quick recovery, our diagnosis of rickettsial and para-rickettsial infections is most likely correct. In the case of slow progress, surely, we are still in the presence of our parasites, but there are missing links helping this proliferation or interfering with the efficiency of our treatment. These links are sometimes difficult or even impossible to establish. Just a reminder of the presence of intra-vacuolar rickettsiae, untouchable by antibiotherapy but seasonally released in the body. Clinical signs of reinfection, also called relapse or reactivation, will follow this.

Further to the use of antibiotics, we add certain adjuvants.

264

The prescription of anti-malaria has been found to improve the symptoms, as well as the biological findings and the evolution of auto-immune disease accompanying rickettsial infections. The results normally take one or two months to become evident. Christopher Columbus described the same positive effects on members of his crew complaining of arthritic pain, who were sucking the bark of a certain tree, the cinchona. Probably by a similar mechanism, the aches of Louis XIV responded to the use of quinquina added to his glass of wine or his coupe of champagne.

Some patients may develop retinal damage, but this complication is extremely rare and can be avoided if adequate control is achieved as regularly as every six months. In any case, this is reversible.

We often prescribe adjuvants, such as vitamin B complex, to assist the possible lack of production of those vitamins by the intestinal bacteria that would normally do so, should the antibiotics have suppressed their existence.

Acidophyllus is taken with the intention of restoring the normal flora of the digestive system. This is particularly important if we consider the wide distribution of a Candida albicans type of condition in patients presenting with any chronic pathological state. Probiotics of dairy origin are to be avoided for the good reason that they interfere with tetracycline absorption.

Cortisone is avoided as much as possible. It works as a brilliant and rapid painkiller and anti-inflammatory. Some patients cannot live without it. Not only does it suppress the immune systems' action, which is very inconvenient when we are in the presence of infections, but also a string of irreversible damage often accompanies long-term therapy.

In experiments on guinea pigs, cortisone has been described as reactivating many old diseases, among them rickettsial infections. In addition, cortisone has been accused of interfering with the diagnosis of rickettsia by lowering the antibody level.

Once more, we would like to create awareness of the numerous publications describing the invasion of our tissues by those intra-cellular micro-organisms, in particular:

- the presence of rickettsia and chlamydia in the cerebrospinal fluid of multiple sclerosis patients (Le Gag, Jadin, 1962, 1986, Sriram, Mitchell 1998)
- the presence of chlamydia in cardiac valves that have to be replaced (Shor in RSA, 1992)
- and also publications exposing that chlamydia and rickettsia not only have been isolated from mitral and aortic valves (Griest in Glasgow, 1963, Drancourt in 1990), but are known to cause endocarditis, pericarditis and myocarditis.
- the publications reporting dermatological pathologies, respiratory infections and the huge gynaecological

impact of those germs, and to use them as a bombscare for those who administer cortisone to these patients, without checking the serological response of their serum against infectious antigens.

Exercise is strongly recommended, and even becomes almost compulsory to maintain the benefit of the treatment. Can we decently ignore our hunter origins and happily buy our food at the local bazaar, pushing it on the wheels of a trolley to the ones of our car. Is the produce of that suburban hunt going to keep us in condition and good shape, as long as the labels of expiry dates are respected?

Rickettsia causes a vascular disease and exercise, properly done, will improve the smooth peri-vascular muscle function, as well as develop the biggest muscle of our body, the heart.

There is also, to encourage the regular use of exercise, the fact that strains of rickettsiae grow better in vitro when they are maintained in an atmosphere enriched with CO_2. This hypothesis will give to exercise a valuable defence argument against the growth of the germs, as it will create a good supply of oxygen, as opposed to CO_2. From this originates the use of hyperbaric chambers, oxygeno-therapy and ozone-therapy.

The suggestion that rickettsiae grow best when the metabolism of the host cell is low, i.e. slowed down through lack of exercise, is another logical reason to get moving.

How do we do this, in our condition?

I know, not easily. But there are many ways. Gentle is the word to start with.

Your muscular cells are inflamed and infected. If you do not give them some fresh air, they will be in such a state from lack of oxygen that sooner or later they may die of asphyxia. On the other hand, if you ask them to function too quickly or for too long, they will rupture, and this will be due to the poor quality of their membranes, which will not allow quick and easy exchange of O_2, CO_2, electrolytes and degradation products. So let's look for something in between no action at all and heavy action. What about sessions of short exercises, like a few minutes to start with, and repeated if you can, two, three or four times a day? When your heart beats faster, you reach your first victory. Stay there as long as you feel comfortable with it.

Was it a mountain? Did you suffer? You see, by being convinced that you have to do it, you can do it. By knowing that it will not take too much time and the energy you do not have, excuses do not stand a chance. A little gives much better results than nothing. Five little alphabetic letters change ordinary into extraordinary.

Now, you are on your way to your next victory: try to reach the point where you glow, or if you feel ready, try to develop a good sweat. This is where detoxification takes place. Your muscles will occasionally surprise

268

you, even for a few seconds, with amazing feeling of tone; your hands and feet will be at more comfortable temperature; your heart will stop having those fast and rough beats.

At this point, you could be ready for prolonging your period of exercises to 10 minutes three times a day. If you are not yet there, do not worry, keep trying — success is around the corner. And there comes the day when your metabolism switches back on. Your muscles are back into curves. You feel better. And you look better.

No real need to increase your period of exercise, unless you have your reasons or feel like it, but it will not be of necessity for your health.

Hot baths are important to eliminate toxins via the skin. After a few minutes sitting in your quite warm bath, the pores of your skin will become dilated and allow the toxins to exit your body in your sweat. These toxins are constituted from dying rickettsial antigens liberated from your cells into the bloodstream under the action of the antibiotics.

So, as you read, the treatment mainly consists of antibiotics.

Is it harmful? Before the advent of antibiotics, infections were treated with poultices made from cow foot emulsified in urine with an extract of orange blossoms added to mask the violent odour. In those days, patients survived their diseases and their doctors' incompetence, thanks only to their strong constitution.

Apart from bleedings and enemas, for those who are upset by the use of antibiotics or other chemical drugs, fire and steel can be used to open an abscess, cauterise a wound or get rid of an infected limb. Nothing is more natural.

Can long-term antibiotherapy weaken your immune system?

Well, in these particular infections, there is not much choice: you or them.

And, without hesitation, your occupants are much more destructive than anything else could be. Also, remember the boost that will be given to your immune system by the increase in the number of circulating germs, due to the good antibiotics.

In fact, the bad reputation antibiotics have for the immune system is a misunderstanding that weakens once more the popular wisdom. Without their help, our immune system would never be able to support us for our present average lifespan.

First, the name itself, antibiotics, means 'against the life'. However, it has a tail: it does not mean our lives, but the ones of our not-so-silent aggressors. Keeping that in mind, antibiotics should actually be rebaptised as being probiotics more than anything else. Nevertheless, that beautiful name has already found a purchaser.

Of course, antibiotics should be used with good judgement, as in fact should any other ammunition, and certainly not against uncomplicated viral infections; the practitioner who prescribes it for any child that sneezes, should get a bad name, not the product itself.

Tetracyclines, in particular, have been accused of deteriorating bones and teeth in children and even adults. This again is such an easy accusation. It will always leave a lasting impression and it is unfair because it is not based on any published scientific observations. In fact, the intake of any chemical might discolour the teeth, especially during development. Far more than tetracyclines, the regular use of sweets and cool drinks, brightly coloured to attract the greedy, might do.

Compared to natural medicines, the real advantage of antibiotics is never highlighted: the antibiotics are subjected to regulations for purity, dosage, preservatives, stabilizers, colorants, while the homeopathic and other so-called natural remedies are not.

They claim to use natural preservatives and sometimes, to use none.

I happened to buy a box of cereal labelled: contains no preservatives. Opening the box later that day, I admired the honesty of those incompetent cereal producers, confirmed by the presence of thousands of worms trying to escape the stringy cocoon. How can one keep a pill as such, without a chemical substrate, called preservative, and without risking it becoming rotten on the shelf in no time, as happens to a carrot in a vegetable shop? Rather the devils I know than the ones of which I still have to discover the unknown side effects.

Human nature sometimes shows a morbid attraction for novelties.

The teratogenicity of numerous chemicals on the foetus has long been known. Yet the drama of thalidomide had to occur before not only the removal of this product from pharmacies, but also to understand the danger of medicating pregnant women.

What is to be expected from practicing a regular intake of vitamins and supplements?

How many potential mutations do they represent, alone or in association? Have they been studied? And how many potential mutations may be sold OTC (over the counter) at the end of every day?

Patients that are on antibiotherapy are seen monthly in our clinic to judge the evolution of their recovery.

Their symptoms are discussed. What can they do, now that they are not bedridden anymore? What about exercises? When are they going back to work? Do they have to still listen to the voice of their symptoms, or can they ignore it now? Should they write exams or wait for the next opportunity? Can she fall pregnant? Is it the right time to immigrate to another country?

It is easy to assess the progress of the clinical picture. So is the decrease in painkillers, antidepressants, sedatives and cortisone that patients are taking.

Depending on each situation, a biological evaluation is performed every three to six months and shows the progress parallel to the other parameters. As reported already to five international congresses, the white blood cells normalise, the liver functions go back to normal, just as do the iron values and the auto-immune factors.

This is what puts me at ease. Because, even if I could brainwash my patients with tender and loving words that would condition them to feel better, as I was accused of doing during the medical investigation, there is nothing I can do subjectively to cleanse the state of their blood.

So I will just keep on publishing — from time to time — these results in figures and numbers.

Based on this assessment, the treatment is prolonged or stopped.

It might take three months, or it may take two years or even more. Eight months constitutes the average.

Patients suffering from multiple sclerosis are advised in every case to stay on treatment for years, if not for life, to avoid or control the reactivation of dormant nests and their irreversible scar tissue.

People suffering from depression are advised not to stop the antibiotherapy before they can live without antidepressants, or nearly so.

The same applies to the corticosteroids in use by

patients falling into the auto-immune system category, and sometimes reduced to function under cortisone for years. These patients are able to diminish the intake of cortisone, very often in an amazingly short period of time. Health is only considered to be back when they can resume their lives without taking cortisone at all.

Often patients suffering from high blood pressure for years are able to stop their antihypertension medication after a few months of pulse antibiotherapy, with no elevation of their blood pressure. The explanation for this could lie in the fact that rickettsial infections are mainly vascular diseases, caused by the invasion of the endothelial tissue by microbes, causing malfunction of this organ and a secondary high blood pressure. So, we are hoping that the discontinuance of antihypertension treatment could be part of our reasonable expectations too.

Eventually, the aim of this treatment is to get us where nothing is required but our own effort and desire to live a serene life, without medication, free of pain and other weariness, with a mind and body coping at a happy level in the human scale.

CHAPTER 13:

MAINTENANCE

"Man's dream would be to be
A passer-by that does not pass away."
—Maurice Maeterlinck—

After the treatment, the disease seems to release its prey, at last. But the patient's recovery leaves scars and sows doubt in his mind. He fears the relapse.

Is he powerless facing this garden all shrouded in night, and this whispering grass where a tireless war between microscopic worlds is always ready to explode?

Where to flee from this net of traps and threats?

What to do with this memory burned by the disease?

Will it be necessary to tack restlessly from one rock of reinfection to the other?

How to carry on in this damned paranoia?

Is there not a little piece of peaceful ground on this

sphere?

There is Antarctica, as we know already.

There, lichens fight a kingdom of snow and ice and ticks are not in sight. The same goes for moss and seaweed. And the same again for the slimy tentacles of the squid. Even if a miraculous louse or a flea in the same state of grace should have landed in the fur of a seal or in the feathers of an albatross, it still would need a series of marvels for the insect to come in close contact with you. It is still true, after this succession of wonders that nobody has ever managed to isolate a rickettsia in Antarctica.

But there is not only Antarctica. There are a lot of lifelines to grasp.

Piles of good books explain how to use them. Exercises, diets, fasting, yoga, meditations are easily reached and very often help. For some, a healthier lifestyle is natural; others will need frequent reminders even about the ABC of good hygiene.

There is no universal panacea for health, or for the joie de vivre.

There is a saying that goes: "One man's joy is another's peril." In other words, there are situations that fat steaks and hiking will not solve. Besides, any thought of steak will probably upset a vegetarian.

Similarly, a session of physical exercise might jam the overexcited machinery of a scientist. In contrast, an athletic body that changes to a sedentary lifestyle will disintegrate quickly, physically as well as mentally.

Obviously these are extreme examples, but how to define the common sense of a mere mortal?

Man, this denaturised ape, nearly healed from his family tree humiliation, has still maintained the profile of an omnivorous hunter. Could he shop at the super-market without seeing the collapse of his carnal but also psychological equilibrium? Does it mean that a human being could do without regular exercise? Then, Churchill, please leave Havana and Scotch, and come and practise some physical training. Lethal result. Lucky, his innate hatred for sport would have prevented such an event.

To live is to be.

But the equation is distorted when we add the word 'well'.

To be well is not the logical result of to live well.

Do exercise regularly, do not smoke or only a little, do not drink or only in moderation, do have a sexual life, but not too much, eat correctly. The purity of biological food is at last regained. Careful, the fanatics of organic health do not lose those so-called benefits by taking nutritional supplements simultaneously, which are unfortunately all chemicals.

There you are, you reach a state of good health, but are you completely satisfied?

Perhaps you are bored to death and in a blind alley. This will do very little to protect you against the intru-sion of a cancer.

Diseases do not always discriminate between people respecting a healthy life and others, before throwing their knives.

Why is this illogical?

Perhaps we are not the maestros of our life, and the care we apply to make it work is derisory compared to the way nature disturbs everything.

Then, what is to be done to help us living down here? How do we protect the collection of cells we are?

Planets also are mortal. And we are biodegradable. We, whose life is carried by matter and whose thought is dependent on chemical transmission. We, the darkest black lighting of all time.

Do we not have any ascendancy over flexible bearings, which would allow us to slow down the time spent on this earth and to move with dignity towards our compulsory death?

Of course, sometimes it may be necessary to change occupation to reduce bacterial contact. Humans are not really here to tame nature. Often, they must come to terms with it.

Obviously, portable phones, radiation, bouts of terror, television, hair dryers and all the satellites running above us do not improve the efficacy of our immune system.

On the other hand, this new chemical invention coming straight from the US will not freeze this aggressive and sordid germ ready to spread out in a new epidemic. Nor will this root extract, as old as Chinese wisdom, update our deficient immune system into a powerful four-wheel-drive vehicle.

Really?

Is there not an essential vitamin or an infallible supplement? An elixir able to repel diseases like the magical potion of Obelix against the Romans?

For example, to add Vitamin A could start a giant rotation of the pointer called health, and bingo, the hell of Dante is opening again. Or indulging a sugar craving will bring in your system enough energy supply to feed those parasitic guests.

This is why I would choose not to go into the sinking sands of the bionetwork we are forming with our germs.

The interaction of biotic factors evolving in an environment without life is the domain of ecology. It is the largest science in biology.

Nature as a whole is dependant on atmosphere, hydrosphere and lithosphere. Factors implicated in the balance between biotic and abiotic are so numerous, so unpredictable and so indefinable. At each moment, they apply themselves to challenge all advice I would attempt to give you on diet.

You could perhaps trust fashion and your instinct for your supplements.

From me, you will get no information, but only the confirmation that your skeleton will be preserved for longer in the ground.

It would be easier to tell you what not to do, like colono-irrigation, taking exit for entries, ozonotherapy that uses our parenteral routes we apply for emergencies only, urinotherapy, which recycles our toxic waste, underwater baby deliveries that ignore our numerous mutations, essentially the one where we lost our ability to breath under water, and many more other attempts for a return to our mother nature.

Besides, where does this trendy slogan come from: 'the natural way', celebrated by the media in the language of our choice. Is it to reassure us against the fear of losing our roots and our identity?

Nature is not beautiful, not ugly.

Nature does not know wisdom, logic and love.

Nature is a constant battle and produces many kinds of cyanides. Rats and their vermin, storms, fires, earthquakes.

In nature, the male covers the female and then leaves her alone to manage the brood, with a few exceptions, unless she has already devoured him.

How can it be confused with a charity?

Magnificent, powerful, wild of course, but not good and not bad.

The world of dreams remains a power as real as your belief in the stars. Your dreams are the engine of your life. They resemble a verbose dogma. But the choice to give shape to those words is, in fact, yours.

As soon as you have decided on your path, you move forwards your chance in the direction you have selected. It will be easy to convince the people around you when the mission is accomplished, and the magnetic field in which you grow will waft you towards your goal, as naturally as any fate would.

There is also the laugh, as irrational as chance, as attractive as Mozart, as obvious as attainable, to improve your immune system. Studies show that endorphins released in the brain, confer on this gesture a value that is scientifically constructive.

Another help against the lameness of our equation 'to live- to be- to be well', is controlling stress. Not the stressful circumstances, but the response to those situations. Stress unbalances our immune system by causing the body to produce hormones that will change the morphology and the action of the T-cells. To see the positive in things, to avoid dark images floating in our minds and to master our brain is a simple question of attitude, and works better than the most refined pharmacopoeia. Indeed all the vitamin C in the world will not make up for a lousy attitude.

And, do not forget to practise the defragmentation of your brain in between all your activities. Open it to any primary beauty you are surrounded by. It could be the voluptuous lips sitting just next to you, the violent spot of colour given by a tree in flower, the wind forcing a dance, the blue of the sky or the roundness of the clouds. Not only does it work, but also it is compulsory for the long life of any computer piece.

Life is a banquet and we, fools, are sometimes starving to death.

Child of the universe, do not cling to your century. You are only short lived because of your choice. Big or small according to your thoughts. Vertical or horizontal, it is only a position. Passing by, but at your own pace...

CHAPTER 14:

RELAPSES

"To die is nothing
To die, what a pleasure,
But growing old… O growing old".
—Jacques Brel—

Unfortunately, one cannot underestimate them. They constitute a daily reality and are similar to the burnt child who dreads the fire. But, their eradication is generally eased if they are recognised as soon as they arrive.

Relapses have two main origins: reinfection from a new source, or reactivation of an old fountainhead.

Rickettsiae and para-rickettsiae have a biological clock: they regain their virulence as seasons change. They are rigorously seasonal diseases.

If I tell you with great embarrassment that tulips bloom in spring and that hens stop laying in winter, it is not the word 'spring' or 'winter' which is going to surprise you, but certainly my embarrassment.

However, if I declare that rickettsiae and para-rickettsiae diseases are seen mainly in spring and autumn, you might have a problem believing me. Or you will politely smile in the face of this new incongruity.

Yet still, we belong to a vital cycle, which governs the cosmos. Though refined, even well advanced, we will never escape this cycle, resembling an exorcism to our occidental mind.

What do we know about those forces pushing our globe? Is it pure coincidence that we breathe eight times per minute, the same period taken for the sea to emit seven or eight waves? Could we be directed by the same control tower?

What can be concluded from autumn suicides?

In Africa, they are called October suicide and they are attributed to the delay of the first rains. But, perhaps more decisive than the drought is the outbreak of rickettsiae at that time of the year and the amount of neurotoxins they dump in the blood stream of patients.

We find another example of seasonal diseases in fish breeding. To optimise the reproduction of those superb Japanese koi, they will have to be supplemented with tetracycline powder in March and October. This is done to control the growth of their Rickettsia pisci, also known in salmon, or perhaps to manage Erlichia rickettsii.

This seasonal outbreak will affect reinfection as well as reactivation.

Ticks, lice and fleas are rife more or less violently according to seasons. So is their infectious material.

Therefore, one has to be protected from their bites, kept away from their contact. Insecticides are sprayed on clothes to repel them. Socks must be worn over trousers to limit access, light-coloured outfits worn to make their presence more obvious, domestic animals are regularly rid of their vermin and thrown off the foot of family beds, children freed from lice, milk pasteurised and meat well cooked, all equally reasonable measures against reinfection.

There remains the reactivation of old and ignored dormant sites.

In addition to the numerous avenues already described to enter our bodies, as if the problem lacked murkiness, there is still one, operating like a public transport. Similar to the Dromadarus called Amoeba or Plasmodium, with passengers called viruses or bacteria, inhaling the toxins of a kind of opium called Rickettsia. Logical to consider that these protozoa, as any other live cell can house and act as a vector for certain bacteria and viruses. This could set off diseases in the host after their release. Those protozoa could destroy or protect the smaller ones from harsh conditions and even favour their growth and multiplication. In return, some protozoa need the presence of bacteria to develop. For example, the plasmodium, agent of malaria, uses bacterial amino acids from the mosquito's gut.

Maintained inside vacuole membranes in the cytoplasm, or forming pseudocysts in the tissues, those multi racial sites are still asymptomatic after-effects of an earlier infection. They are not even formed by ancient veterans as they escaped bombardments by antibiotics, gastric juice aggression and the hostility of antibiotics, thanks to their protective membrane.

This observable fact, well described for the gondi parasite, responsible for toxoplasmosis, is called endodyogenicity.

Similar conditions could apply to many germs having in common a slow growth, such as tuberculosis, syphilis, rickettsia, chlamydia, mycoplasma, borreliosis, malaria, brucellosis, bilharzia, babesia, leptospirosis, yersinia...

In fact, symptomatic diseases are less frequent than asymptomatic diseases. The capsule of those cysts, as well as the membrane of those syphilitics' gummas or the caseum found in tuberculosis, is resistant to antibodies, antibiotics, pepsin, hydrochloric acid, etc. In these conditions, the micro organism may stay alive and multiply slowly for years. The rupture of the membrane will cause a relapse or a reactivation of the disease.

The impact of this process could be local: i.e. when in the presence of a sudden onset of eye tumour, brain tumour, or myocardial infarction, commonly called heart attack, as it was not the result of a degradation process.

The crash could also be general: this could explain perhaps a man suffering from multiple sclerosis who suddenly loses the use of a limb and is confined to a wheelchair, while another comes back with an acute attack of rheumatism or also the development of other auto-immune diseases, such as a crohn patient who has almost forgotten his illness and urgently needs surgical intervention.

Another good example of revival of infections in different organs and at different stages is illustrated by the syphilitic gummas, that can burst in the brain of a patient considered as cured many years after the primary infection, and explain the sudden and unexpected dementia.

Similarly, malaria could re-attack its victim 20 years later, taking advantage of a new weakness in the immune system, such as a chronic leukaemia.

How could the germs remain dormant? How could they be permanently frozen in that form?

To start, a census will be necessary.

Unfortunately, cystic forms do not have the same antigenic surface as the free form. Thus, the biological diagnosis does not exist. Then, we are left with no other choice but to be ready for this event.

The excess of stress, the potent viral diseases, the close

contact with chemicals, the radioactivity could ignite this reactivation.

The important factor is to recognise the enemy as soon as possible and to reduce it to silence once again.

Luckily, this task is less difficult than in the first infection, because the immune system, trained by the previous antibiotic action, remembers as much as the patient does.

But sometimes, the awakening is fulminant.

For this reason, the treatment should be to administer at least a few times a year, and this for life, to chronic patients with biological and clinical evidence of major systemic diseases, without awaiting relapses.

CONCLUSION

"Nothing is done of what we still have to do."
—*Napoléon Bonaparte*—

The disease exists.

A secular entity that takes on so many faces according to its different fields of conquest and evolution levels.

The diagnosis is possible.

Not belonging to any routine investigation, it stagnates in the medical subconscious.

The treatment is available and efficient.

It does not kill. It only needs a few more definitions.

Even though infection is not the cause of every disease, it is omnipresent and therefore can interfere with each vital cycle. The importance of these facts in our daily medicine is not to eliminate death, but to displace it. Death is nothing but a later version of birth.

We will give back our body, but not at 20 and not all broken down. Not under the infectious yoke, but only when it is worn out by love, exhausted by pleasure and satisfied with work. Not with the wind in its feathers, neither the foot on the accelerator, nor swirling eyes full of stars. But turned white by our successive triumphs and wrinkled under the weight of dignities, we will lay down our arms with our gnarled fingers. Good night, we will say respectfully, bowing for the last time to our unrecognisable and magnificent patriarchal faces. Releasing slowly the reins suddenly too heavy.

Facing our destiny, we will accept rest. This is our sagacious friend who has waited many years to lay out our fatigued body and allow our overloaded memory to unfold at last.

Conscious of the name and shape of our predators, we will recognise them more easily and we will break free as often as necessary.

For one cannot eliminate them.

Charles Nicolle's dearest dream was to see the destruction of germs as the ultimate means to eradicate human diseases. Eventually he also had to accede to the impossibility of the mission.

Then, we have to live with our parasites, endlessly putting them back in their place and foreseeing their mutations.

To achieve this, it is not enough to unmask a few parasites in a book and to stand as the champion of a group of scientists from the Pasteur Institute, even if they were bright.

It is not enough to bring up to date a mass of colossal

but forgotten researches.

Nor to moan about discrepancies in language, in cultural barriers and other misunderstandings regarding some disclosures.

It is only a first step. I have done it, believing it was necessary. I stop here.

Call me if you wish to continue...

GLOSSARY

agglutination — the clumping together of bacteria caused by the introduction of antibodies to such cells. In the Micro agglutination test, we introduce non-virulent strains of rickettsia, the antigen, to the serum of a patient. If the serum agglutinates, it means this serum contains antibodies. Therefore, this patient has been exposed to the germ.

antibody — a protein substance produced in the blood or tissues of animals or human in response to specific antigen. Antibody reacts with or neutralises that antigen.

antigen — any protein substance that causes the body to produce antibodies to counteract it. Bacteria, toxins and foreign blood cells are antigens.

apoptosis — programmed cell death. Normal part of development and maintenance.

arteriopathy — disease of the arterial wall.

arthropod — invertebrate that belongs to phylum Arthropoda; has a hard skeleton, a segmented body, and paired, jointed appendages.

attenuated form — germ, which has lost, permanently or not, its virulence, its ability to cause disease in a host.

binary fission — equal division of a cell in two; a type of asexual reproduction.

carrier or vector — healthy person or animal who carries a germ but is immune to the disease and transfers it to people or animals.

cardiolipin — in some auto-immune diseases, an auto antibody is produced again this phospholipid and could increase the risk of vascular thrombosis in the patient.

Carpel Tunnel Syndrome — weakness of the hand caused by the median nerve compression.

Cartesian — having to do with Rene Descartes methods: a philosophical system resting upon his famous axiom Cogito; ergo sum (I think; therefore I am) seeking to impart to metaphysics the certainty and precision of mathematics.

Catatonic Syndrome — increased muscular tone from various origins.

cavity — in tuberculosis infection. Necrosis (caseation) of the lungs may empty into bronchi with resulting 'cavitation'.

Celiac disease — is a disorder characterised by malabsorption, abnormal small bowel structure and intolerance to gluten.

Charles Bonnet Syndrome — visual or olfactory hallucinations due to affective disorders, mainly seen in elderly people.

Chinese Restaurant Syndrome — overuse of sodium glutamate, causing headaches and nausea.

Crest Syndrome — auto-immune disease related to sclerodermia.

Creutzfeldt-Jakob Syndrome — rapidly progressive type of dementia from viral origin.

Cri-du-chat — type of mental retardation.

Crocodile's Tear Syndrome — tears pour from affected eye with eating. Occurs after recovering from Bell's palsy.

Crohn Disease — or regional enteritis is a chronic inflammation of the ileum (small intestine) from unknown origin.

Cruzine — extracts of Trypanosoma cruzi showing anticancerous properties.

cytoplasm — see protoplasm.

dormant forms — see attenuated forms. Those forms are more likely to be found in cysts or intracytoplasmic vacuoles.

ecology — a discipline of biology that studies the interrelations among living things and their environments.

electrolyte — substance that dissociates into ions when dissolved in water. Electrolytes balance between the extra and intra cellular liquid is strictly regulated to maintain a normal metabolism.

endemic — stage of a disease, when it is regularly found among a particular people or in a particular locality.

endocarditis — inflammation of the smooth membrane that lines the cavities of the heart.

epidemic — rapid spreading of a disease.

gumma — granulomatous inflammation associated

with tertiary syphilis. Could involve any tissue, are usually painless but could be very destructive. Rare after penicillin treatment.

leucopenia — abnormal decrease of white cells or leucocytes.

lymphocyte — see Reticulo-endothelial system.

mitochondria — structures found in the cytoplasm of cells, which produce most of the energy and oxygen required by them.

myocarditis — inflammation of the muscle part of the wall of the heart.

pandemic — disease spreads over an entire country or continent, or the whole world.

pancytopenia — abnormal decrease of white cells, red cells, platelets in the blood.

phagocyte — a cell capable of absorbing and destroying waste or armful material, such as disease-producing bacteria. The absorption and destruction of this material is called phagocytosis and was first described by Metchnikoff, 1908 Nobel Prize for Physiology. Metchnikoff was a disciple of Louis Pasteur and the tutor of Charles Nicolle.

protoplasm — early biologists thought that the cell consisted of a homogeneous jelly, which they called protoplasm. Today, the name cytoplasm is used and means part of the cell outside the nucleus.

reservoir — substratum where a germ will survive and grow. A reservoir could be a human being, an animal, biological products like milk, meat, cotton or dust and water. Reservoir could be the source of infection directly or indirectly via a carrier.

reticulo endothelial system — a system of cells in the body, especially in the spleen, lymph nodes, bone marrow and liver that function in freeing the body of foreign matter and disease germs in the formation of certain blood cells i.e. lymphocytes involved in the recognition of antigens and production of antibodies, phagocytes, etc.

saprophyte — organisms living on decaying organic matter i.e. moulds, mildew, bacteria, etc.

Sjögren Syndrome — dry mucous membranes (eyes, mouth, etc) associated with rheumatoid arthritis.

thrombocytopenia or thrombopenia — abnormal decrease of thrombocytes (platelets) in the blood.

uveitis — inflammation of the uvea.

vector — see carrier.